A MAP FOR THE JOURNEY:

Living Meaningfully with Recurring Depression

by Nan Dickie

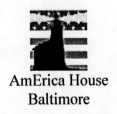

AmErica House
Baltimore

First printing

Library of Congress Cataloging-in-Publication Data

Dickie, Nan
  A Map for the Journey: Living Meaningfully with Recurring
Depression — 1st edition.

ISBN: 1-58851-107-3
PUBLISHED BY AMERICA HOUSE BOOK PUBLISHERS
www.publishamerica.com
Baltimore

Printed in the United States of America

Disclaimer

This book is sold with the understanding that the author is not engaged in rendering psychological, legal, or other professional services. If expert assistance or counseling is needed, the services of a competent professional should be sought.

Dedication

I dedicate this book to my nephew, Mike Beckner, and the many, many other young adults who are coming to terms—and learning to live meaningfully—with recurring depression and other mood disorders.

What is required of us is that we love
The difficult, and learn to deal with it.
In the difficult are the friendly forces,
The hands that work on us.

Rainer Maria Rilke

Acknowledgments

It's much easier to find the right words to develop a character or express an emotion than it is to adequately acknowledge people who have supported me on my journey to the completion of this book. To do it properly, I have to go back many years.

My family has played a vital supporting role. I am grateful for the support of my brothers and sisters, especially for the ongoing loving care of my sisters Marcia and Betty.

Charlotte Braithwaite, my "best friend from Grade 8," believed in me at a time when I had no idea who "me" was. And she got inside every word of this book as it was taking shape to make sure it was exactly the word I wanted in that particular spot.

I'd like to acknowledge my longtime friends Ruth Decary (who has shown me what courage is during her chronic illness of 30 years), Barbara McKay, Evangeline Kubin, Barb Galeski, Kate McCrone, and Martin and Barbara Rumscheidt (who helped create the title for this book).

Soon after I was introduced to a medication that allowed me to function adequately, I began to seriously examine my life. Psychotherapists Rhona Rosen and Mal Weinstein helped me sort out many of my temporal difficulties and chart a course for a more fulfilling life.

My wonderful soul-friend, Jean Taylor, with whom I have walked thousands of miles on Sunday mornings, is always with me though she has moved half way around the world.

Ingrid Pacey, my psychiatrist, has seen me through many episodes in the past 12 years, and those episodes have been more bearable because of her consistent care. Dr. Ron Remick has adeptly guided my medication regimen for several years.

Earlier versions of many of the articles in this book found their first airing in newsletters of the Mood Disorders Association (MDA) of British Columbia. Had it not been for that organization, its Executive Director Robert Winram, Editor Bill Gibson, and the responses I've received from many thoughtful readers, I would not have had the courage (or is it nerve?) to offer my thoughts and feelings to the wider world.

I was spurred on in my efforts to write this book by two friends who, by writing and publishing their own books, showed me the way and gave me the courage to write mine: Wendy Thompson, who taught me the discipline of writing before breakfast, and Marja Bergen, who shares my illness.

Finally, but first, there's my partner of 12 years, whom I call MP. This book would be nowhere without MP's love, perseverance, patience, encouragement, and the odd push to press me on.

I have many people to thank for my life, particularly those who have believed in me when I didn't think there was anything to believe in.

Although I feel utterly alone in the darkest stretches of my depressive episodes, with the awareness, understanding, and care of friends and loved ones, I am, in truth, not alone, never alone.

Annotated Table of Contents

Section 4: Since You Asked

There and Back
*Jess candidly tells Emma what an intense
depressive episode is like* 195

Dare to Ask
*How do you ask questions of someone who
gets depressed? What is appropriate to ask?* 205

Asking about the Worst
Devon asks Andrew about his worst fears 211

Appendices

Special Pieces for Supporters
*Articles and stories of special relevance
to family and friends* 219

Suggested Reading List
Further readings on depression 221

Useful Internet Resources
Some websites that are useful to us 223

Glossary
An explanation of many terms used in this book 225

Index of Pieces by Theme
All pieces sorted thematically for easy reference 231

The Beginning

Foreword

I am a psychiatrist in private practice with a primary interest in psychotherapy. More than 12 years ago, I met Nan Dickie, and she became my patient. She chose to see me because she wanted to be treated psychotherapeutically as well as with medication for the depressive episodes she suffered.

In the late 1960s and early '70s, when I was a young medical student and psychiatry resident, I developed a deep interest in the psychodynamics of mental disorders and in psychotherapy. I believed, naively as I later discovered, that psychotherapy could cure all psychological ills.

As I moved from residency to private practice in psychiatry, I learned, of course, that this wasn't so, and that for many patients with recurring depression and other illnesses, medication was either the primary treatment, or a necessary adjunct to psychotherapy. Unfortunately, while drug therapy was crucial for many patients, there weren't many choices of medication at that time.

When I first met Nan, she already knew she had a depressive illness. She had been taking an anti-depressant for several years, which had helped provide her with significant, albeit not complete, relief from the devastating depression that at times engulfed her.

As Nan and I began our work, we explored her family history, her formative years, and her life as an adult. It became apparent that depression had been part of her life from very early on, and in due course, she came to more clearly understand her life, and resolved various troubling events she had experienced.

Despite this resolution, her depressive episodes continued, and we both came to realize that medication was an essential part of preventing and treating what we came to understand as illness.

Both Nan and I found it difficult to accept the reality that her type of depression is, in fact, a primarily biochemical illness. But we did accept it, and we began our journey to explore new medications, developed since the early 1970s, in the hope of preventing, or at the very least ameliorating, her episodes. In the course of this exploration, psychotherapy has played a supporting role and will continue to do so.

In the twenty-first century, doctors have many classes of antidepressants to prescribe. Many medications are also available to augment the antidepressants, including mood stabilizers to prevent extreme ups and downs. But the work of understanding and treating this illness is painstaking and ongoing. Doctors and patients, working together worldwide, continue the gradual process of unraveling the subtleties involved in combining these medications to give the best results and the fewest side effects.

Although the medical community's sophistication and knowledge about, and treatment of depression has advanced, we must never forget the person behind the illness. Our patients have families to care for, and talents to offer. They have work lives and communities. They have souls to nurture as well as bodies, and the former, their spiritual dimension, may need tending as much as the latter.

This book goes to the heart of all these dimensions. Nan reminds us all—doctors and patients, friends and partners, indeed anyone who seeks to understand this illness—that treating depression successfully requires a conscientious, multi-faceted approach.

Nan has a special, remarkable skill; she is able to be both a compassionate participant and a perceptive observer. After years of reflection, she has much valuable advice to offer. She tells us how to catch the early signs of recurrence, how to avoid denying that an episode is under way, and how to move quickly to treat symptoms early. She gently reminds us to be alert to the effects of adjustments in medications, to treat ourselves with compassion, particularly when in an episode, and to always remember that an episode will end even if it feels like it never will.

Nan takes care of her body. She takes care of her soul. She communicates clearly and openly with her partner, her family, and her friends. She asks for help when she needs it. Her book reminds us that all of these measures are crucial to living well with recurring depression—as they are crucial to a healthy life for any of us.

This highly readable book offers valuable understanding to anyone interested in recurring depression. Above all, it will provide sustenance, solace, and support for those who live with this illness, and for those who care about them.

Ingrid Pacey, MD, BS, FRCP(C)

Introduction

The title of this book probably raises several questions for you. Your first question understandably may be: What do the words "recurring depression" mean?

If you identify yourself as a person who experiences this type of depression, your next questions may be: How can I live more meaningfully with the abrupt and lengthy interruptions in my life? How does the "map" I live by differ from other people's maps?

If you do not experience recurring episodes of depression, you may be asking yourself: How can I best support someone (sister, son, partner, parent, friend, or acquaintance) with this illness?

If you ask any of these questions, this book is for you!

Types of Depression

Everyone has experienced depression at some point in life. It may have been precipitated by a sudden loss (of a child, partner, or job), by an abrupt change (moving to a new city or country, having a baby), by prolonged stress, or perhaps by long-term financial insecurity. In any case, it may well have been caused by an external event.

A single incidence of depression is enough in one lifetime for a person to say, "I've been there, and it's a rotten experience."

But many people endure repetitive episodes of an even more desolate type of depression. This depression is characterized by darkness, isolation, and despondency.

Visits here may be as regular as clockwork. They may occur every winter. Depression related to the amount of sunlight available is called Seasonal Affective Disorder, or SAD.

At times episodes of depression are part of a cycle that spans manic highs and devastating lows. This is the pattern of the illness known as manic-depression, officially called bi-polar mood disorder.

For a lot of people, depressive episodes strike at no particular time, prompted by no apparent external factor. This illness goes by various names including depression, uni-polar mood disorder, and, historically, melancholy. Various forms of treatment, from medication to psychotherapy to electric shock treatment, may or may not succeed in alleviating the cruel symptoms brought on by this illness.

This latter type of depression is the perspective from which *A Map for the Journey* is written.

This illness manifests in episodes of depression that occur, unwelcome and generally unpredictably, again and again and again. In all cases, it presents the sufferer with deep pain and formidable challenge, and can, if not acknowledged and treated, ruin any hope of a satisfying life.

A depressive episode may go on for weeks or months, and abates according to its own strange, incomprehensible timetable.

There is Good News

In spite of this bleak picture, one can live meaningfully with this disorder, not merely cope or deal with the illness, but live a full and long, if bumpy, life.

A life that includes recurring depression may not be one of success or happiness as normally defined. The "ground" on which an individual who experiences recurring depression creates and nurtures life is vastly different from that on which other people find themselves. The terrain is at times gently rolling, as it is for other people, but it also contains unique, dark regions with deep and dangerous holes. The underlying assumption of *A Map for the Journey* is that one can traverse this rugged ground with meaning, purpose, and satisfaction in spite of periodically tripping into these pits.

Maneuvering through successive depressive episodes is not like any other endeavor. With this illness, we may enter the Perilous Pit over and over again, only to discover that the way through the ordeal is different each time. And the necessary means by which we do that are often difficult to discover, and seemingly impossible to execute. Indeed, sometimes the most effective action is non-action—that is, a dose of self-compassion, patience, and faith that this dreadful episode will pass before too long. In a depressed state, it is very difficult to summon up these resources.

An Unusual Map

A Map for the Journey attempts to be exactly that—a map to which readers may refer in order to understand many of the issues, problems, concerns, and yes, joys that people with recurring depression encounter as they journey through their lives. My intention with this map is to focus on many of those issues, offer support, suggestions, inspiration, and possibly some vital relief to those who know this life all too well.

About the Author

I know the map well. I have visited all the places described in this book. I have experienced recurring episodes of depression for the past 40 years, since my early teens. During my episodes (which vary in length, but usually last from four to eight months), I experience the characteristic despair, discouragement, isolation, fear and exhaustion that the illness provokes.

In the past several years, during my well times, I have sought to understand the disorder better, explore new ways to meet the challenges of my down times, and record the pattern of my cycle from wellness, down the slippery slope to desolation, the long, hard climb up from "the pit," to full recovery.

About four years ago, in an attempt to understand and portray the immensity of a depressive episode, I wrote about several of my experiences in point-of-view pieces and short, short stories. Twenty-eight of these pieces have been published in consecutive issues of a newsletter for people with mood disorders. The response to my writing has been enthusiastic, and people ask for more. Hence, the notion of a book was born.

Who Would Find This Book Useful?

A Map for the Journey is written primarily for those of you who experience recurring depressions as I do. But its audience is in fact much broader. This book can be very useful as a resource to support groups for people with mood disorders, in day houses where groups of people are trying to come to terms with the illness, in hospitals where individuals are being treated for particularly bad bouts of depression. School counselors, social workers, the pastoral ministry, and psychotherapists will find this book useful in their efforts to understand the complexity and substance of this life. Counselors may recommend the book to their clients and patients as a means of alleviating the horrible sense of isolation and hopelessness experienced in a deep depressive episode.

Finally, this book will be of significant interest to those of you who are family members or supportive friends of people with depression, who wish to understand the trials of people with a uni-polar mood disorder, and to support and nurture us as much as possible.

A Few Building Blocks

A Map for the Journey rests on several important assumptions:

- The illness is illogical, irrational, erratic and uncanny, and is based largely on faulty brain chemistry;
- One of the greatest challenges for us is to acknowledge and accept the fact that we have this illness;
- We continually try to work through life's situations knowing that we will at times succeed, but often falter, and sometimes fall on our faces;
- Though we face unique stumbling blocks, despair, and disappointment, we are still worthwhile human beings, and our lives are more and larger than our illness;
- New medications resulting from ongoing medical research will improve treatment for recurring depression;
- We must always choose life, in spite of it all.

Other Resources

Fortunately, in recent years several helpful books have been written about depression, some by people who themselves experience recurring depression. Bookshelves offer autobiographies of famous, and not so famous people grappling with the illness. A number of self-help books and guides and more formal books addressing medical aspects are available, as well as works that offer valuable inspiration to those of us who contend with the reality of this illness throughout our lives.

Many of these books are listed and described in the Suggested Reading List at the end of the book.

A Map for the Journey is not intended as a substitute for, but rather takes its place beside these other resources and offers a unique insight into this difficult life.

Making Your Way Around and Through This Book

A Map for the Journey is a "reader-friendly" book. Jump around it as you wish or need from article to story to poem to graphic display. You can refer to the Annotated Table of Contents, where a short explanation of each piece is included to help you zero in on what is most relevant to you at any given time.

If you choose, you can read the book from cover to cover, as it is logically divided into four main sections reflecting the different stages of experiencing and living with recurring depression. In short:

- Section 1 outlines the common early experience with the illness, including articles with useful information and strategies and stories of hope and inspiration;
- Section 2 offers pieces showing further experience with the disorder and ways in which various characters have refined their lives, given the reality of their illness;
- Section 3 presents several pieces of reflection and spiritual considerations linked to our common lives, and outreach possibilities;
- Section 4 answers many of the questions you may have been afraid to ask someone who experiences episodic depressions, even if that someone is you.

I hope this book will address your particular needs at many points of your association with the illness of recurring depression.

Section 1:

Recognition and Learning

Symphony in Words

I have often likened my cycles to the seasons. When I am well, it feels like summer time. When I am entering an episode, it feels like the life is seeping out of me, just as the leaves loose their hold on the trees in the autumn. The depth of depression feels not unlike the depth of a prairie winter, except the light is so bright in prairie winters, and there is no light in the cold darkness of depression. Spring is a time of renewal, of new promise, of hope, which results in new growth.

The following poem expresses my sense of the seasons in my life with recurring depression. It reminds me that "what goes down always comes up," and that good mental health returns over and over again.

Music fills the halls of my soul
And takes me far away
To familiar places and happy times
Of our concordant past.

* * *

The song is now soft
A happy melody of summer green and blue.
Staccato notes reveal the fast-beating heart
Of a new surprise.

The rhapsody spills out its tale
A prelude to an unborn score.
The theme is here and now, and we
Ask questions. (What's it all about?)

September brings a melancholy tune
Of winds whispering in the trees
Asking of me things I wish to hide.
The dance becomes confused
On the waves of forceful music.
O God, where is that summer song?

And, now, the winter march
That carries heavy, cold, dark notes
Into the very core of my being,
Casting aside the memories of earlier times,
Drowning out the hopes of future songs.

But, suddenly the horrid march is stopped
And music of a struggling soul puts forth
A quiet effort to build itself a home.
Oh summer, you have brought your warmth to bear!

The song escapes itself
And reaches out to touch the sky,
To feel the earth,
To sense the songs of other souls,
To find some harmony among all else,
So it may know its freedom and its place.

O music, Music, please flow free
And try to touch a corner of their hearts,
Giving of yourself your love, your song,
Delivering to them that which swells inside.

Not a Straight Path

Since you are reading these very words at this very minute, you are probably somewhere on your path to knowing and accepting the fact that you have the illness of recurring depression.

Maybe your eyes are three-quarters closed and you are trying to pretend you really aren't reading this. Or perhaps you are reading this on the bus, on your way to work, where everyone around you can see that you are reading "that kind of book."

Whatever the case, you are somewhere on the path between denial and acceptance, between hating yourself because you believe that your problems are obviously all your own fault, and being at peace with yourself for having courageously accepted your illness and its challenges.

You and I had no choice about the fact that we are on this journey. We may have inherited genes that cause the disorder. Or our brains just decided to do something out of the ordinary. And we certainly didn't create the prevailing attitude of the society into which we were born, wherein compassion and understanding are all too scarce. What a start! But we do have the choice between denial and acceptance of our illness. And if we do choose acceptance, we do have choices about what we do with and about our illness.

What lies between our place of origin and where we are today?

There are many different answers to that question because there are so many of us. But there are some common signposts along the way to tell us how far we have moved, and how we are faring now.

Let's take a regular like-you-and-me sort of person who experiences recurring depression. I'll call her Lauren. This is what her path looks like.

Unawareness and Denial

For Lauren, as for many of us, this unchosen and turbulent journey began in unawareness. Her high school years were a painfully bumpy, up and down time. The alternation of elation and despondency perplexed, worried and frightened her.

When she completed high school, she hoped (indeed, decided) that these feelings would never return.

But in her early twenties, the amplitude of her highs and lows became even greater.

Am I sick? she asked herself.

No. She couldn't face that fact. So, she chose to vigorously deny it.

I'm not sick! I just have to grow up and get past these childish moods.

Lauren swept her secret under the carpet.

Awakening

By the age of 24, Lauren's denial scenarios were losing their power.

They were necessary and natural when I was young, but not any more. I've got to find out what's going on, and figure out how to fix it.

She finally went to a doctor. He told her, in no uncertain terms, that she had uni-polar mood disorder, which, he added, "is a legitimate mental illness."

Bargaining

Finally, Lauren reached a point where she could admit to herself, and to herself only, that she had an illness.

She tried to bargain with the illness, with the horrid intruder she called the Ominous Presence. She got married, had kids. She would live happily ever after.

There. All I really needed to do was get married. Problem solved!

Self-blame

Alas, after five years of everything to do with marital bliss, which proved false, Lauren couldn't bargain any more, and took up self-recrimination.

If I hadn't been an idiot for being so competitive in high school, I wouldn't have got depressed. I shouldn't have got married; I should have just been a career person. I have brought this whole stupid affliction upon myself. What a moron!

She was thrust, or more accurately, she thrust herself into a strangely different kind of depression, wherein she felt the victim of her own screwed up mind, body, and soul. She finally admitted what she had tried so hard to deny.

I'm unhealthy, repulsive, and abnormal. I'm mentally ill.

Like others struggling as she was, she was not "just" depressed. The earlier stages, which she hadn't really dealt with, came to bear. She was mired in a devil's brew of denial, self-blame, and bargaining. She was retreating into the worst sort of "blended" depression.

Anger

After a while, Lauren grew tired of the worn-out "I am a despicable person. No wonder God hates me" tape. So had her friends. Some of them had given up on her.

She got angry. Not just angry but hostile. She struck out at the world as if it was to blame for her condition. She raged at society's depiction of people with mental illnesses as poisonous freaks. She cursed her parents for her problem, for her differentness, for her pain. "Why did you even have me?" she cried bitterly.

Eventually, exhausted, she fell silently despondent. She became increasingly isolated and was even contemplating giving up on life itself.

Her dearest friend from childhood, Karyn, had said to her gently a few times, "Lauren, I really believe that some talking therapy would help you sort this out. It helped me a lot. Please, give it a try."

Finally, with no other recourse, Lauren took her friend's advice.

It worked for Karyn, and it couldn't possibly make me feel any worse.

Acceptance

In the course of the next two years, Lauren would more than once curse Karyn for her stupid idea.

For what seemed an eternity, she spent a great deal of energy and money in therapy with a sympathetic counsellor. Through the painful and gainful therapy with her counsellor, she came to accept, with no denial, no bargaining, no self-blame, and no anger that she had what her doctor had announced many years ago, a mood disorder.

What a relief! No more fighting with herself or anybody else any more.

She heard about and joined a support group and developed some comfortable friendships with people who experienced life much as she did. She discovered that most of the members of the group had gone through similar trials, some shorter, some longer, some more painful, some less. The consensus was that the journeys were necessary and necessarily personal, and that there was no easy formula and no instruction manual.

Integration

Lauren had acquired a brand new feeling of lightness, rightness. She began to discover, as she accepted her illness "to the bone," something even greater than acceptance. At the ripe old age of 38, she found a wonderful feeling of integration, of wholeness. At long last, the words honesty, integrity, and true-to-self became relevant to her. Though she knew that she would most likely experience more episodes of depression in her life, she felt she would be capable of meeting the challenge.

Now she could address other important issues like finances, career, and family relationships. Now she could get on with her life.

Lauren had done it. She had "arrived."

She was showered with valuable insights to do not only with her illness, but her life in general. They felt like bonuses, rewards for a job well done.

Finally, finally, finally! Now I can use my mental energy productively. I can really live when I am well, and I can learn, more and more, how to care for myself when I'm not so well. The whole process has been worth it.

Heart Talk

Angela is like everyone else who says sometimes, "My head tells me to do this, and my heart tells me to do that."

But it isn't that simple for Angela. It doesn't end there. She's trying to figure out what's going on inside her head. It's pretty hard to understand some things when you don't share them with at least one other person. It's hard to put words to a thing when it is so huge, when it is so "in your face," that you can't get a proper perspective on it. It's like when you stand so close to a big picture on the wall that all you see is colours all mixed up. Well, it's something like that.

Angela wants to figure this out for herself. The last time she went to the doctor, he suggested that she take a new anti-depressant. But she wasn't into pills.

"They don't solve problems," she said sternly. "They just cause side effects."

So recently, when things went a bit strange again, she decided she would work it out on her own. What she noticed over a period of a month or so was that her head was telling her to do this. Which was fine and ordinary. Then her head began to tell her to DO THIS, and there didn't seem to be much room for her heart, or anything else, to say anything.

A message that Angela heard two weeks ago was, "You are a worthless person. You haven't done anything with your life. Look at you. You're empty. There's nothing to you."

She wondered where that came from. Life had been going along all right. She thought she was pretty happy with most things.

But she considered the question seriously and concluded that her mind was telling her these things.

But why should it be doing that when I have a happy life? she asked herself.

She decided that the logical thing to do was to counter this negative message with a positive one, and tell the negative message to get lost. So she tried. But she found that the part of her trying to counter the negative message was sounding very weak.

Why should that be? I'm usually pretty good at pulling myself together. Maybe I haven't been loud or convincing enough.

She tried to be more definite with her counter statement, but it just got lost in thin air. The message, "You are a worthless person," and the rest of it became much louder, until she couldn't hear the counter argument at all.

I'm usually disciplined enough to steer the course of my thinking. Why is it not working now?

After a while, the negative messages multiplied and became intolerably loud.

"Would someone please turn the stereo down!" she cried. But who could turn the stereo down? She was the only person who was living in her body. And it was her head that was full of loudness.

All of this was wearing Angela down terribly. It came to the point where she was receiving nothing but negative messages. She came to believe that she was indeed a worthless, rotten person. Her mind was giving her so many good reasons.

"You've never set any goals for yourself."

"You've never carried through with any plans you've made because you're so lazy."

"You can't do anything well, especially your job, especially anything."

"You'd better act well, because that's the only way to show people you're okay (which you aren't)."

On and on it went relentlessly. What could she do but believe? There was no countering. The messages reached volume 10 in her head.

One day it taunted her, "You can't even tie your shoe laces properly."

That statement triggered something in Angela. She had just enough sense left to realize, or at least hope, that that statement was false. She decided to tie her shoelaces to prove the point. She put her runners on, untied. She looked at the laces and became extremely nervous.

What if I can't do this? Then I may as well give up.

At that point, a quiet little message made its way into her mind, amidst the horrible negative stereo clatter.

"Hello, Angela," it said, softly but distinctly.

It wasn't really a voice that said hello to her. It was a signal coming from somewhere, from somewhere other than her mind. It was so quiet that Angela almost didn't hear it. But she did hear it. She did!

She closed her eyes, letting go of her assignment to tie her laces, and listened carefully.

"Hello," she responded quietly, a bit embarrassed that she was doing so.

Another quiet message came to her, "Hello Angela, this is you heart. Not your physical heart, but your feeling heart."

She felt weird, but put her hand over her physical heart. She sighed because it felt good. It felt like home, where she hadn't been for a long time.

"Angela," continued her heart, "I know you haven't been able to hear me because of the stereo noise. But I want you to know that you are alive and well in here. The problem is that you have an illness, and that illness is blaring in your head now."

She thought that she was going a bit crazy. But her heart message was so warm, so convincing, so supportive, that she decided to listen for more. So she remained still and kept her attention on her heart.

"Angela," her heart went on, "Please believe me. It is an illness that is giving you all those negative, untrue messages. Those messages are not of you, they are symptoms of the illness. Do you believe me? Do you understand?"

Angela didn't know what to think. But for the first time in months she felt somewhat at home with herself, that her heart and spirit were not dead in her after all, and she decided to go with the heart message.

"Yes," she said definitely, and after a moment, "So what should I do?"

"You need to have the illness treated," her heart responded. "You may need medication for it, or therapy, or both."

"But I've done the pill routine, and it didn't work," she replied coolly.

"You have tried only one medication," her heart firmly replied. "You have no idea what other medications are available that may help you."

Angela had to agree that her conclusion was based on a sample of just one medication.

"Yes, but," she found herself saying. "Yes, but..." being her usual response of late to any positive idea from any source. "Yes, but, which other medication? How do I find out about it?"

"Maybe it's time for you to trust someone," her heart said.

Damn it. How does it know I don't trust anyone?

"Okay, I believe you. You're right. I haven't trusted a soul about this."

She was silent for several moments, then asked shyly, "Do you..., do you think you could help me work this through?"

"I would be very pleased to," said her heart.

"Where should I start?"

"First thing you must do is go back to your doctor," her heart replied emphatically.

So Angela went back to her doctor to begin working out how to find relief.

It was a long road with plenty of false starts and bumps, but with the right amount of a new prescribed medication, and some useful therapy, the clamor of the illness receded, and her heart and spirit took centre stage again, where they belonged.

She still hears the loud, tormenting, stereo noise once in a while, because her illness isn't simple. It isn't a one time affair. But Angela now manages her illness much more successfully and tries always to listen to her heart.

Snapshots from a Trip

I feel so <u>well</u> these days, these months. I can hardly believe I ever get depressed. The only thing reminding me of my mood disorder is the medication I take daily. Ah, well. I'm happy. Life is treating me well. And I, it.

↓

Something is going on. My mind feels a bit confused; I must try harder at work. Maybe this new task is beyond my capabilities. But that doesn't make sense: they <u>loved</u> my last project. And I enjoy my job a lot. My relationship is fine. I'm not fighting with friends. What's happening in me???

↓

I don't want to go to any social events these days. I guess I want more quiet time now. <u>Or</u>, have I offended everyone? People look at me strangely. Things <u>were</u> going so well. What do I have to do to be happy again?

↓

OH, HELP. I'M PLUMMETING, BUT I DON'T KNOW WHY. IS IT THE SEASON? I FEEL ISOLATED WHETHER I AM ALONE OR WITH PEOPLE. MY HEART IS HEAVY, MY BODY TIRED.

↓

This is getting worse, and worse. I'm such a loser. What ever made me think people liked me? Dumb.

↓

This is hell. I feel dirty, ugly, invisible. I shut myself away at home. I sleep all the time. I am a zombie again. My doctor increased my pills. Maybe death would be preferable. Oh, shut up.

↓

And when the cycle ends, I arrive back where I started and know it for the first time.... The light coming through the trees is beautiful. I'm so glad I'm alive. I look only forward now to happy tomorrows...

↑

I feel renewed in a way. Life is worth living again. Where have I been for so long? It was <u>such</u> a waste of time, that down.

↑

I made my first meal in months today. I got together with Kerry for a walk. It was almost fun.

↑

Could this possibly be new light, new hope I see? Can I trust it? Can I <u>not</u> trust it? I will, I <u>will</u> trust it!

↑ ↑

Stand up. Fall down. Stand up. Fall down. Stand up...	Over and over. Again and again and again.

↑ ↑

It's such a slow and steep climb now. I'm <u>so</u> tired.	I don't think I have the energy to do this. Not now.

↑ ↑

I'm in that deep, dark, cold, horrid pit, tormented by the Ominous Presence. Have I ever been anywhere else? I am trapped, sentenced, exhausted, less than nothing. I can't think straight. I'm ashamed and embarrassed, so I hide in silence. I am in despair, dread, seeing impending doom. Days are excruciatingly long. I have never been other than totally depressed in all my life. I am paralyzed. I brace myself for the torment I cannot prevent. It screams at me, incessantly. Turn it down! Turn it off! No one can do that for me. There is no hope.

AWOL

It was Saturday evening. Great! Carmen was so looking forward to her and Brian getting together with Peter and Sandy. They had all been pals for years and hadn't seen each other for a few weeks.

The plan was to have houmous and bread and wine at Brian and Carmen's place, then go out to their favourite Greek restaurant for the main course, followed by dessert at Peter and Sandy's. Perfect plan!

They'll be here in fifteen minutes. Carmen hustled to get ready. *I'm so eager to tell them about my new job, and about the kayaking weekend Brian and I just had.*

The doorbell rang.

She went to answer it. Suddenly, she didn't know what to say to her guests.

Do we have a hug at the door? What will I do with their umbrellas? What are the house rules anyway?

She was in a bit of a panic. This wasn't like her. She had been well for months now since her last episode. What was going on?

"Hi, Carmen," exclaimed Sandy. "Great to see you!"

Yeah, but I know they're happier to see Brian than they are to see me, Carmen found herself thinking.

"Don't worry about your shoes," Brian said.

But we always get people to take off their shoes at the door. Brian is trying to suck up to our friends. Carmen was shocked by her own thoughts.

"Come on into the dining room," Brian invited.

I'm usually the one who does the inviting. Brian is horning in on me, and I don't like that.

"How's the garden?" Peter asked.

They're only interested in Brian, the gardener. We have a lovely garden, and Brian gets all the credit, as usual.

"Can we take a look?"

They're just rubbing in how wonderful Brian is. No one praises the assistant, the one who makes the meals, carts the dirt, buys the bricks.

41

"Great walkway."

So maybe I bought the bricks, but Brian, of course, laid them, so he gets all the accolades. I have nothing to show for myself. I may as well not even be here. I wish I were a "product" person. Instead, I just read and write, and look after Brian and work. I'm a "process" person, an assistant, never the principal. I'm tired of this. I've got to change.

"Good houmous," Sandy said as they all dove into the appetizer. "This is fun. Thanks for the progressive dinner idea."

It was my idea a few weeks ago to do this, but, of course, they think it was Brian's. Why isn't he giving me credit now?

Brian and Peter and Sandy found all sorts of things to laugh about.

What's so funny? All they ever do is laugh. Why aren't people ever serious? They try to humour me, and it doesn't work. I'm stone-faced. I'm not in the mood for jokes. I want out of here. I can't stand this.

"Time to go to the restaurant, hon," Brian interrupted Carmen's negative, spiraling thoughts.

What have they been talking about? Have I embarrassed myself? I certainly haven't really been here. I wish I weren't.

Carmen thought about her sorry state of mind in the car on the way to the restaurant.

"Things okay?" Brian asked with some concern.

She didn't want to let on that she was having difficulties.

I'll snap out of it any minute now.

"Oh, I'm okay. Just tired, I guess."

She knew if she said one word about how she was really feeling, she would lose control and either break down and cry, or yell out in frustration.

How long do we have to spend with these people? We haven't even had dinner and I've had enough.

"Are you going to have your favourite dish?" Brian asked, as they perused the menus.

What makes him think he knows what my favourite dish is? Actually he does, I have to admit. But am I that predictable? Well, I'm not going to be.

"No. I'm having salmon."

"Great choice."

Damn it. Why does he always have to be so agreeable?

During the dinner, which seemed, to Carmen, to last forever and a day, she kept her eyes low, on her food. She felt embarrassed, even ashamed. She knew she wasn't "at home."

Why is this happening to me now? I was so looking forward to this evening, and now I'm hating it.

Finally, finally, the get-together was over. She felt horrible. Brian knew something was wrong, but after ten years of being together, he knew enough to wait for her to say something. She was tempted to let it all out and bash herself about.

After all, it's my own fault. Instead, she wisely said, "I'm going to bed; I've had enough of this day."

With her head on her pillow, and her thoughts safely to herself, Carmen tried to figure out what had happened when she went to open the door to greet Peter and Sandy.

This has an awful feeling to it. It's too much like the beginning of a downer, but I was feeling fine until...Boom! Am I in trouble? Oh, help!

She felt like crying. But instead, she decided to let go of the evening, to not worsen the situation, and see what the morning would bring. This was a tactic she had learned several episodes ago.

In the morning, as she was awakening, Carmen quickly did a check.

Am I here, or am I as absent and negative as I was last night?

Much to her surprise, after checking all her inner corners, she knew that she was absolutely here; she was fine.

What was last night all about? she wondered. *Will I be okay now?*

She couldn't allow herself to feel too optimistic, because mornings were always her best time of day.

Carmen never knows the answers to her questions when these incidents occur. Sometimes events like this are the start of terrible trips to hell. Sometimes they are just blips going nowhere.

Well, I may have been absent without leave last night. And I don't know about the rest of today or tomorrow. But right this minute I am present.

She sighed, and got up to begin her new day.

Spilling the Beans

I am usually very careful and deliberate in deciding whether to tell a new person that I have a mood disorder. I think about my relationship with him or her, consider our level of trust and confidence, and how I would feel if they didn't keep the story to themselves.

This is a self-protective mechanism, and I do not apologize for it. I have been disappointed more than once by telling an unsympathetic soul of my disorder. Each time this happens, I recoil and withdraw, and it takes time, energy, and courage to "come out" again. Hence, I take great care.

This time I didn't. It just came out.

I was at my monthly chiropractic appointment with Dr. Rowan. I had been receiving treatment from her for a couple of years and felt very comfortable chatting about anything. Well, almost anything. Even though she is a medical practitioner, and skillfully adjusts my body, I had chosen not to say anything to her about my faulty brain chemistry. After all, what does a mood disorder have to do with my fifth vertebra?

But this day I was brimming, because an article I had written on mood disorders had just been published by the Depressive and Related Affective Disorders Association (DRADA) at Johns Hopkins University. Dr. Rowan knows that I have had articles on other topics published, and I had even shared a few with her.

Midway through my treatment on this day, I was very relaxed and feeling safe, as usual. Before I had a chance to contemplate what I was about to say, I proudly offered, "I've just had an article published by an association at Johns Hopkins University."

Oh, my God, I had taken that irrevocable now-you've-done-it step. Since I am not one to lie, I couldn't follow up with something like, "It's an article about the big toe." So, nonchalantly, I continued, "I wrote an article on mood disorders. Did I ever tell you I had a mood disorder?" It had the ring of a confession that is a daily event.

Without missing a beat (and why should she?), Dr. Rowan said, "No, I don't think so." I tried to continue the conversation sensibly, though part of me was in panic mode.

When Dr. Rowan had finished my treatment, I glanced at her face, trying to read it without being obvious. Was she looking at me askance? No. Does she now feel sorry for me? I don't know. Can she hardly wait to tell others? I doubt it.

She was her usual self. I still felt a bit tongue-tied, and I knew if I tried to explain myself with my "I'm-usually-more-deliberate" line, I would trip all over my words, so I changed the subject.

I had a few days to reflect on that experience. What did time do to my concerns?

Well, I am sure I can trust Dr. Rowan. I trust that she won't think less of me because of my disorder. I am sure I will receive the same quality of treatment I always have. And I know she will treat the information as confidential.

Why do I have such a strong need to hide my secret?

That's easy to answer superficially. This disorder is not well understood by most folks, and some people pooh-pooh it with comments such as, "Just pull yourself up, girl. We all get the blues, you know."

But there are more subtle and harmful reasons for hiding, which finally I have been able to bring to the surface.

Try this one. If people know I have a mood disorder, they will see what a despicable and rotten person I am, how dark, poisonous, and ugly I am to the core, they will label me weak, useless, and deficient. That is my mental reality, over which I have no control, when I am in a depressive episode.

No wonder I usually choose safety in silence.

I am not suggesting that I ought to tell everyone I meet about my disorder. I must gauge the appropriateness, value, and risk of each situation.

Unfortunately, every time I deliberately choose not to tell a special person of my disorder, I am cutting out the possibility of their understanding me better. Their picture of me is inaccurate and incomplete. They can know me only partially and don't have a sense of my whole being if I leave out this major part of my life story.

Contrary to my fears before disclosure, it seems that when others gain this new insight, they do not see me as despicable, dark, and poisonous. Rather, they seem to see me as a courageous individual who has a special struggle with life, who at times needs compassion and love, and at other times encouragement and levity.

The burden of depression is lessened a tiny bit when I share with a new person the fact that I am a depressive. It does not make the illness or a particular episode go away, or even lessen the pain; but in disclosing I do feel more integrated (though flawed), honest, and cared for.

Next time, I think I will spill the beans on purpose.

I'm So....

Following are the entries covering a four month period from
Brenda's journal:

I am very enthusiastic about my new job. All my skills are being
tested: interpersonal, technical, organizational, and writing. I will
interview clients from a large organization, design a series of
manuals, and work with a new state-of-the-art software package.
This could be the break I've been looking for. When I've completed
this project successfully, there's a good chance I'll be up for
promotion.

I interviewed our client's Personnel Manager today. The interview
went well, and the client said I had been very thorough in my
questioning, but now I'm having a bit of trouble getting the
information from that interview down on paper. Maybe I'm just
nervous about this challenge, this chance to move ahead.

I must remember to double-check my work before I give it to my
boss. I made a grammatical error—just a small one—but he
wasn't too pleased. Yes: I must double check all my work.
Double check. I've made a note of that.

I've been putting in quite a bit of overtime lately,
because I need to make sure I'm covering _everything_
properly. I'm getting tired of this overtime work, but it
has to be done. I have to do it.

Well, I've finished the interviewing stage of this project,
thank heavens. It was getting difficult for me to do. It got to
the point where I wasn't phrasing my questions very well.
Maybe I'm not a great interviewer after all. I'm sure the
design phase will be easier. It's my favourite stage of this
sort of project.

49

I started designing the first manual this week. Why am I having trouble with it? This work has always been a breeze for me. But now my thoughts aren't clear at all. This is so frustrating. Maybe this project is just too complex for me.

> My boss told me—in a kind way, almost sympathetic—that maybe I need help with my project. How embarrassing. But what could I say? I *am* having trouble doing this work. So now Robert is helping me. But I find it difficult explaining to him what this assignment is all about. This isn't like me. To tell you the truth, I feel *really* embarrassed.

This is ... *awful*. Now Robert is in charge. I just couldn't put it all together properly. I can hardly blame my boss for this move. This isn't like me at all.

> *I am so humiliated...* I'm *off the project...* I couldn't even *assist* Robert properly. In fact, I made a serious mistake in an aspect of the design of this manual, and *he* got in trouble—not me. I feel like going into hiding.

> Sick leave. I thought I was embarrassed *before*. I can't blame my boss for insisting that I take sick time; I feel fuzzy in my head. I really feel ashamed.

I decided to go to my reading group tonight. I decided I would concentrate really hard and focus so I could follow the conversation. It didn't work at all. I couldn't participate in the discussion because I couldn't connect one person's sentence to another's. I feel so inadequate.

> This *can't* be an episode. My mood is okay; my physical energy isn't bad. But my mind is *terrible*. I'm getting more confused about things every day.

I talked to Jane today. Well, *tried* to talk. I was no where. So was my mind. I wouldn't blame them if I got fired.

This guy at the grocery store thought I was drunk. Just because I'm muddled and befuddled. It took me three times longer to do my shopping than usual.

I boiled the kettle today. I mean boiled it *dry*. Remembering notes not helping. I never can find them anyhow.

I thought I loved cooking. But this *bloody* spaghetti.... The package instructions doesn't make sense. What to do? They make it so hard.

I don't want to see *anyone* now. Probably forget there names.

This is making me mad—
or is it angry? or something whatever

I wonder if their talking about me at coffee brake.

I dunno. What did you say? How am I supposed to...?

I'm so... I'm so... I'm so *what*?...Oh, yeah, ...dazed? Is that it?

Wake up. Take pills. Remebember.

Typings to hard. Spell badly. To hard to write too.

No tv. No radio. No chatting. Just trying to do each day very simple.

This is to hard. I'll be back when I am doing more better. Till then....

Brenda didn't write in her journal again for three months. When she began to emerge from her episode and to re-unite with herself, she wrote this poem.

It's Safe to Emerge
You hide away where none can see
And nudge and poke and pester me.
Your existence is assured
Though my vision is obscured
By the wall you are behind
In the fortress of my mind.

Too many years have passed us by.
You never seem to want (or try)
To let me know just who you are
Though we've never been too far
apart.
What are you doing to me
By forcing out <u>this</u> poetry?

You've never told me of your name,
Or more important, what's the game?
Are you shy, or is it fear
That keeps you hidden? I want to hear
Your story—tell me right out loud,
Then I will blow away the cloud
Of self-suspicion; a question mark
Will no longer face me in the dark.

But wait! How could I be so bold
To want you standing in the cold,
Naked to the eyes of them
Who seem adept at taking pen
In hand to find <u>their</u> hidden parts,
Expressing feelings from the heart?

So, stay inside and grow and find
Words that will give me peace of mind.
Be what you are, but come to me
And, on your own, I hope you'll see
That you've got reason to be proud,
To declare your feelings right out loud.

One month later, Brenda wrote another poem.

A Reminder
Hold on to these when things are down:
Staccato notes, expansive sky,
The yet-new knowledge of the I
that is (not of the I to come).

The search continues as the day,
Though the night may hide its stars.
Please dwell not on the times in dark,
But on the now, the happy heart.

To find a pleasure—tis so new—
In daily or in weekly acts.
Where has your mind been all this time
That you have missed the living facts?

What is it? Let it happen,
Let it come; oh, let it be.
And maybe in so doing
You will find the long-lost "me."

By the end of the next month, Brenda was feeling very healthy once again. She was back at work, visiting her friends, and cooking spaghetti successfully.

53

Don't Take a Vacation

Every now and then I contemplate taking a holiday from my pills. Well, actually, I don't get that close, but I find myself thinking the thought.

And then I get really scared.

I have come a long way from that wreck in the late seventies who was flailing around in the ocean of lostness. I can recollect it clearly—so clearly in fact that I fear being sucked right back in again. Depression is only a wave away.

I have been maintained (mostly successfully) on an anti-depressant for twenty years—first with a tricyclic, and now with an SSRI. During this period I have, with my doctor's approval and guidance, cut back on my medication a few times.

You ask, "Why? If it ain't broke, why fix it?"

Well, I am a minimalist. If I can function as well on less, then I would rather take less. I am not certain what physical effects these medications are having on my body in addition to restoring my mood, so less is better—at least that is my logic.

I have not been very successful in cutting back on my medication over the years, though I have insisted upon trying, repeatedly. Fortunately, I have, in general terms, come to the "right" dose with my doctor. The dosage varies over time as my brain chemistry changes. Sometimes we have to experiment.

Each time I have cut back on my medication, I have tried to convince myself, "I can live with fewer pills; it's mind over matter." Then, within days, my mood, in spite of my best intentions, may darken severely. I become uncharacteristically insecure, painfully sensitive, and remote from everyone. I find myself face to face with the dreadful feelings that warn me a full-blown depression is about to occur. Without consciously choosing to, I blame everything else in my life for my feelings: I must be in the wrong work. I really hate my partner. I'm a rotten person. I analyze everything but my pills.

Bravely, or, to be more honest, foolishly I march on. For a few long days I torment myself mercilessly. I can't remember ever having felt well, and my universe shrinks to a poisonous ball.

Finally, after I've had enough of this spell in hell (and one day of it is too much), in desperation I return to my regular dosage of medication and wait impatiently to start the agonizing climb. I do have to wait, as anti-depressants take many days, even weeks, to work, and that time seems excruciatingly long.

Why do I insist on putting myself through this avoidable pain? Why can't I just accept, and let it be?

As I've said, I am a minimalist. But this is not the whole story.

There is, deep in me, a place of denial and doubt that I really have a physical problem. How many well-meaning family members and acquaintances have said over the years, "You don't need pills. You just need to pull yourself up by your bootstraps," or words to that effect? This can be a very compelling argument to a person who is despondent, isolated, feeling helpless and hopeless.

So I have, too often, and too readily, agreed with them. After all, I am an intelligent, healthy person, living a happy life with meaningful work. And I feel "normal," like other folks most of the time. Why should I need pills to balance my mood? Aren't I strong enough to deal with life the same way everyone else does?

Well, the fact of the matter is: yes, I am strong; but no, I am not able to function properly at all without anti-depressants. My brain chemistry is faulty. Period. I am similar to the diabetic who requires daily insulin to keep alive. Plain and simple.

This bothers me immensely. I hate being humbled like this, knowing I am not self-sufficient.

I also hate to admit that I at times have doubt. Not rational doubt, but undermining fear doubt. Doubt about the medical profession. Do they really know what they are talking about? Doubt about my assessment of relatives and acquaintances. What if they are right about the bootstraps?

If I admit my dependence on a certain drug, I face frightful questions. What if I develop a tolerance for it, and there isn't another one on the market that will work at all on me? I have developed a tolerance for one drug, but I was successful in switching to another, more current one.

What if I am stuck in a remote place, have run out of my medication, and absolutely cannot get any more? I always pack twice as much medication as I need on a holiday, plus an extra prescription, but that does not eliminate all my fears.

What if I was in an earthquake (a real possibility where I live), my pills were destroyed, and I couldn't get to a pharmacy?

These are for me very terrifying and realistic questions. I do have faith in medicine, that there will be another possibility for me, but what if there isn't? What if...? I feel very vulnerable. But I am not a victim.

So, in an attempt to avoid contemplating horrendous possibilities or to escape terrible feelings of doubt, at times I have chosen to pretend that I don't really need medication. In an effort to prove I am not vulnerable, I have chosen to deny what is real.

Dependence is not easily accepted by one who has enjoyed independence in most aspects of her life. Being handicapped, or challenged, or whatever, is tough for one who has been gifted in some ways, and capable in most.

Horrendous possibilities, vulnerability, dependence, being handicapped. These are extremely difficult things for me to accept willingly. But, unless I do, I could find myself walking down that bleak, black, senseless road of denying myself pills again.

I don't want to. It's not worth it. I can't afford it. So, I try to accept.

How Could They Possibly...?

It was a very unusual bunch of folks, to say the least, who were gathered at the far end of the field. It was a warm spring day, with a light breeze—perfect conditions for personal bests on the cinder track. Athletes in this meet had already broken several international records in the past five days.

The competitors lining up for this final race were each as nervous as the other. They had all come a long way to this final of the combined men's and women's 100-metre sprint at the Unusual Olympics. Each of the athletes reached this final through local, provincial, and national qualifying meets. No other runners imaginable could have more poignantly represented each area than these final five hopefuls.

"Runners ready," called the starter. Hearts pounded in the chests of the racers. They proceeded to the starting line, being careful to remain behind the chalk line. The starter waited patiently.

In Lane 1, Nicole, a middle-aged professional artist whose rise to fame had been meteoric many years ago, was poised in her wheelchair. She had been in a terrible car accident eight years ago, which made these wheels her legs for the rest of her life. Incredibly, her arms and hands had been spared injury and her love of her art more than made up for crippled legs and related limitations. But Nicole was now facing another harsh reality, the worsening arthritis in her fingers and wrists. She feared she would never be able to paint again (painting had been her only great love in life), nor wheel herself around on her own much longer. She was fiercely independent and couldn't imagine having to depend on others for her mobility. How could she possibly be in this race?

In Lane 2, Kent was trying to keep his heavy-as-concrete legs moving. His heart and soul were in anguish, and his mind tormented him mercilessly. He was in another of the incapacitating downs of his mood disorder and was always at the mercy of his unpredictable brain. This horrific episode had been going on for months, and Kent couldn't remember ever in his entire life having been in any place other than this absolute hell. He could barely concentrate on where he was, let alone imagine placing one foot in front of the other time

59

and time again to get to the end of the track. He struggled to the starting line. How could he possibly be in this race?

In Lane 3 (the so-called "fast lane"), Jill, at the peak of her lengthy running career, was stretching her long, strong legs, taking deep breaths of fresh air, stealing one last moment of silence to centre herself mentally. She was used to this pressure, but there was much, much more than usual riding on this race. Jill was about to attempt to break the longest-standing world track record. She was completely confident of her chances, and she could almost taste the fame and fortune of her future. But this was absolutely her last chance, as there was an age limit for the Unusual Olympics, and she was one week away from it. She looked around at her competition. How could she possibly be in this race?

In Lane 4 was a young, brilliant woman, Candace. She was a Rhodes scholar whose mission was to become an architect so she could design and then supervise the construction of state-of-the-art housing for the blind. Her prospects were excellent, or at least they had been until she had contracted AIDS from her husband. She didn't know which would be the hardest: to die without fulfilling her mission, or to accept her husband's infidelity. Both were dreadful, and terminating, realities. Her health was declining rapidly. In her despondency, she had come alarmingly close to committing suicide more than once, and as recently as last week. She was spent physically, emotionally, mentally, and spiritually. How could she possibly be in this race?

In lane 5, Slim, who was anything but, looked around at his competition. "This'll be a piece a cake," he bragged under his breath. His cockiness was offensive, and apparently unwarranted. Just two weeks ago he was full of self-contempt, had the energy of a slug, and couldn't think straight. But this was different. He was "up," which meant uncontrollably manic. Nothing and nobody was going to stand in his way, not even the celebrated Jill. He hadn't run a race in his life or ever even donned these stupid runners until the trials for the Unusual Olympics. Slim was a good 40 pounds overweight and smoked a pack a day. But he knew that he was going to leave the competition in his wake. How could he possibly be in this race?

"Take your marks!" With their various encumbrances, each racer approached the starting line. They poised themselves, as well as they could, behind the chalk line in readiness for the starter's gun. They looked towards the finish line. It seemed impossibly far away for all competitors except Jill, and, of course, Slim. "I'll probably get there after dark," moaned Nicole, though it wasn't yet noon. "I'll be there in a flash," Slim announced boastfully.

There was a brief stillness in the bleachers and on the field. Then... "Bang!"

And they were off!

The crowd watched enthusiastically as the athletes expended every ounce of energy they could muster to hurl their variously-endowed bodies down the track. Nicole, with great concentration and pain, shoved the large wheels of her heavy chair with her disfigured arthritic hands. Kent tried desperately to concentrate his tormented mind on the task at hand, to put one concrete foot in front of the other, again and again and again. Jill chased the world record with unparalleled conviction and determination. Candace, so near death, gasped for each breath and tried to suppress those omnipresent thoughts of suicide. And Slim, who had thought he was Superman, obstinately ignored his body's capabilities (or lack of same) and remained ridiculously convinced that he would win.

In the bleachers, some fans were cheering for their favourite athlete, some fans cheered for all the athletes, and some fans turned away, feeling a bit nauseated, mumbling they had to go to the washroom.

No one had ever seen a race like this. But, then again, this was the first ever Unusual Olympics. All the other events were finished by now, but hundreds of spectators had waited in line for hours this morning, just to see this final. Everyone knew well ahead of time that this was going to be the race of the decade.

After what felt like an eternity to four of the athletes, but to Jill just a flash, they were within 10 metres of the finish line. With their super-human desire and exertion, the competitors reached the finish line, and lunged across, utterly exhausted.

At the end of this race-to-end-all-races, every one of the runners but Jill collapsed. It was too close to call a winner.

Competitors and fans alike waited in silence to hear who had prevailed.

An excited voice finally came over the loudspeaker. "Ladies and gentlemen: As you can imagine, the race was a photo-finish, and the photo has now given us the results of this race! You will not believe this! For the first time in the history of track and field, we have a dead heat, or perhaps we should call it a "live heat," of **all five competitors!** Each runner crossed the line at precisely the same instant as every other runner!" Jaws dropped. The voice paused. "And, ladies and gentlemen, we may well have a new World Record! Stand by!"

None of these great competitors, save Jill, had enough energy to even hear the loudspeaker. Slim, who only a few minutes ago knew he was absolutely unbeatable, felt emotionally and physically crushed, and had plummeted into hell. As for Nicole, Kent, and Candace, they didn't care who had won. All that mattered to each of them was getting across the finish line sometime today. Jill, breathing easily, was resting on her own on the grass and strained to hear that she had performed her miracle. It felt to her as though she had literally flown down the track.

When they were sufficiently rested to be able to think again, the four exhausted runners moved slowly, and with immense effort, to get off the track.

Each of the four felt a strange shift within their aching bodies and fatigued minds. It was unmistakable and deep-seated, this shift, and each competitor strained to grasp its meaning. They had all, these unusual four, received an important message. During this greatest run of their lives, each runner had reached a catharsis.

Nicole, the artist, resolved that she would take up storytelling (it's creative, and she won't have to use her arthritic hands doing it). Kent, in spite of his acute depression, felt a profound shift from his constant depressing truth of "I can't" to an affirming "I will." Candace realized deep in her soul that she would never kill herself, no matter what. And Slim decided that, although he had yet again been an victim of his manic-depressive illness, he would no longer flog himself for being sucked into unrealistic expectations.

The loudspeaker broke the exhausted silence. "Ladies and gentlemen: I have an important message. I'm sorry to report that Jill missed the World Record by 1/1000ths of a second."

Jill was visibly devastated. She closed her eyes and reflected for a moment. Then she humbly accepted her defeat with an uncharacteristic feeling of peacefulness, which surprised her immensely. Endowed with this, *her* catharsis, she sprung up and jogged over to celebrate with the other competitors.

This unusual race had been, for each of its competitors, a challenge of self-acceptance, of doing the very best with the stuff of life, be it hardship or gift, that each had been given. Each runner had exhibited extraordinary courage—the capacity to move ahead in life and accept its consequences in spite of despair, loss, and hardship.

The unusual five crowded atop the podium to receive their gold medals with enormous, and well-deserved joy. Each of these exceptional individuals had reached beyond any conceivable grasp and had achieved inner and outer greatness, in spite of it all.

Two Days

Tuesday

It's going to be a great day! I'm not even finished my coffee and already I can feel the energy.

It's been the usual old seesaw, up one day, down the next. But today, this—THIS—is solid excellent health. My episode is gone, gone, gone. Finally! Only good days from now on.

The water feels so good. I could swim forever. Even after the long walk. Or maybe because of. Must be the endorphins. The drive-over-and-swim-two-laps days are history.

A full hour! How long since I've done that? Doesn't matter.

I should be tired. I'll likely feel the muscles later, but I'm loaded with energy, and my mind's so clear. Perfect for woodworking.

Good thing we don't need that extra storage space immediately. My blanket box has been on hold for eons. But I'm making progress today.

Musn't try to make up for lost months in a single morning. Hard not to when you're on a roll. But woodwork's good for that. It's so...What?...Painstaking, that's it. You just can't rush wood. Push too fast and you can almost hear it say, "Enough already. Isn't it lunch time?"

Even my usual salad and cottage cheese were extra tasty. So's the tea. Feels good to put my feet up and relax. I was right. My legs are telling me that they've been exercised, not really sore, just there. Give them a break. Drive to the store.

I'm having a ball tossing stuff into the cart. Last week I hated it. Felt closed in, smothered. Couldn't find half the stuff on my list. Haven't had to use my list today. Don't need it. Well, maybe I'd better check just to be sure.

Yes! I knew it. Got everything we need. Maybe a bit more than we need. A few frills and treats. Why not? On a day like this it's important to "go with the flow."

It's early. Lots of time to unload the car, have my nap, and mow the lawn before dinner. There goes the phone.

"...Oh, Steph, I'm sorry, but I really do need my nap... No, I feel great but it's like a necessary habit, you know...Yeah, even on good days. Sounds great. Let me know okay...Yeah, and thanks for keeping an eye on me. I need all the help I can get... 'Bye, and Steph, I really am sorry I can't go just now."

Boy am I sorry! Wonder what goodies I'm missing. Don't even think about it. Just go and lie down. Honestly, sometimes this nap business seems like such a waste of good time.

Not today! One, hour, almost to the minute as usual, and I'm fresh and alert. What a privilege to wake up twice to such a gorgeous day!

The new-mown lawn smells so sweet. The flowers are brilliant. The leaves are winking at me. Can't be dew at this time of day. It must have showered while I was sleeping. Such a beautiful garden. I feel so blessed.

What'll I do about dinner? Are you kidding? After that shopping spree? A gourmet feast, that's what. And a smashing dessert for Pat and Chris later.

It'll be so good to see them. How long has it been? Four months since this blasted episode started. Four, very long, unsocial months. There's a lot to catch up on. So, we'll just sit out here and gorge ourselves on crepes and catch up.

What a day! Perfect except it was so short. Oh well, tomorrow's just a sleep away. I can hardly wait.

It's so difficult to imagine ever being ill. It feels so distant, yet it's been so recent...

Wednesday

I'm so groggy. As if I didn't sleep. But I did. Did I swim too much yesterday? Couldn't swim today to save my soul. Maybe the grey day is getting me down. Who knows?

Have to get out of here. I'm feeling closed in. Walk to the cafe or something. It's not far. Maybe I could manage. They don't mind if I stay and rest there. Makes it look like they have business.

Too tired to walk. Have to drive.

How long have I been staring out the window? About half an hour probably, ever since I got here. Usually I read a chapter in that time. Not even a page today. They must think I'm nuts.

Something I'm supposed to do on my way home. Pick up stamps? Shampoo? What is it, damn it? I just want to go home. I'm hungry.

I eat the same old stuff every day for lunch. Why can't I remember now? The fridge is a blur. Nothing makes sense. I have to eat something. Toast. I can do that. Butter. That must be what I forgot.

Oh well. Toast and jam is okay without butter. Where's the jam? Tea would be good. That's easy. Good thing the toaster shuts off and the kettle whistles or I'd probably burn the house down.

I know I have to expect good days and bad days when I'm getting better, but this is hopeless. Actually it's dreadful, that's what it is. Dread is the worst. My mind's so fuzzy. I was so sharp yesterday. It was yesterday, wasn't it?

I could have my nap. It's too early, but I'm so tired. A long nap. Yes, then the day won't seem so long.

Can't sleep. I'm so alone. I'm scared. Get up. Go to the library. There're always lots of people there. I won't be alone. If I try to read, I might even doze. That would be good. They don't seem to mind.

Okay, take my pill and then go. Did I already take my pill? I took the morning pills. The slot in the plastic box is empty. But my afternoon ones are all in a bottle. I'm quite sure I didn't take it. This is so embarrassing, even just to me. Fortunately no one else needs to know about it. Better get another plastic box. Write that down.

Now I can't find my car keys. I've looked everywhere. I want to cry. Why can't I? I can't stand it here. I'll have to walk.

Still cloudy. Where's my jacket? In the car?

It is, and the keys too. May as well hang out a sign, "Car for Theft." Not very funny really, but pretty good for a day like this.

So dopey. Shouldn't be driving. Be really extra careful.

The guy behind me blasted his horn. How long has the light been green?

"Pardon me, Miss. Sorry to wake you, but your book's going to fall."

So, I finally did get some sleep. Maybe only 20 minutes but better than none.

What was I supposed to get on the way home? I didn't write it down, so lost it somewhere in my thick brain. Why don't you make lists, dummy?

I suppose the garden's nice. I can only say that because I remember that yesterday I was enthralled with it. It's just a smear of colours now. Too much work to face.

Dinner. A drag to make. I'm alone tonight. I hate dinner alone. But, with nobody watching I can get away with peanut butter and jam. That's about the best I can say for being alone. Truth is, if I had anything planned, I'd cancel. That doesn't make sense. Nothing makes sense.

I'm so trapped in my head. It's been such a long, dismal day. Didn't get anything done. So, why am I so tired?

I can't remember what "feeling good" is like. Not one single solitary clue what it's like.

Please let me sleep. Please let tomorrow be better.

Note from Nan:

This is a realistic two day period in my recovery from a depressive episode. Though I am uni-polar (I experience depression but not mania), I have sometimes felt I must be bi-polar because of how "high" I feel some days when I am recovering.

This great feeling is due in part to the fact that, during my down time, I forget what normal life is like, and I am reminded on the happy days during my recovery that good health is such a blessing, and much of life is a wonderful gift.

A Very Special Blessing

December is a very busy time of year in Blue Joy's home. It's time again to create, select or assemble, wrap, pack, and distribute a present to each and every person in this whole wide world who wants one, and that means a lot of presents.

Contrary to popular belief, Blue Joy's parents have 100 offspring, not just a bunch of elves. Mom and Pop need all the help they can get to carry out their colossal responsibilities to the huge population south of their Arctic home.

There is one thing distinctive and very special that happens each year at Blue Joy's home that you may not be aware of. You see, a child was born in each year of the first century of Mom and Pop's marriage (except in the years when there were twins, in which case they skipped having a child the next year—thank heavens, for Mom). On each centenary of a child's birth, that child has the privilege of giving an additional present to people he or she has selected who have a direct or remote connection to his or her very own given names.

To give you an example: sister Lily, the 86th child, gave an extra present to each of her designated folks in 1986 (and 1886, and 1786, and all the way back to the beginning of time, it seems). Lily chose to give presents to everyone whose name had something to do with flowers—to everyone named Rose, Iris, Ivy, Holly, Flora, and so on. In 1886, she gave each of them a unique, opaque, beautiful vase. In 1986, she gave all her floral people a gold lapel pin with their special flower on it.

Blue Joy's favourite sister, Gemma, the 45th offspring, gave the additional present of a precious gem in 1945 to all the folks whose names had to do with gems: Ruby, Di, Pearl, etc.

Just to ensure that everyone receives an additional present in each century, twins Cracker and Cookie, the 99th and 100th children, offer angel food cake to all the unfortunates who inadvertently fall between the cracks.

Now, Blue Joy, the 96th progeny of Mom and Pop, was born on one of those oh-so-rare February 29ths. Because of this uniqueness, Mom and Pop gave Blue Joy the distinct honour of bestowing a very special blessing upon her chosen people. As you know, blessings are more valuable and precious than mere presents. A present is usually a concrete thing you can see and touch, whereas a blessing is an invisibly significant benefit or favour that gives happiness to its recipient.

So, the year 1996 was an exciting year for Blue Joy. It was once again her own year to choose an unforgettable and exceptional blessing for each of her selected people.

Blue Joy dreamed about this wonderful time of blessing for many years beforehand.

The first question she faced was, "To which fortunate folks will I give my special blessing this century?" In 1896, she had chosen all the people in the world who were full of joy at that time. Unfortunately, that was not a busy year for her, even though it was the middle of the "gay nineties."

To be sure that she would make a wiser choice of beneficiaries this time, Blue Joy decided to consult Gemma. After putting their heads together for a year or two, Gemma exclaimed, "Hey, sis! I've got the perfect idea. Blue is not only a colour, it's a way of feeling. Why don't you give a very special blessing to people who sometimes feel blue?"

"Great idea, Gem. Thanks!"

Blue Joy thought about it and decided that the specific blue people she would bless were those who were polar, just because she herself had lived at a polar address all her life. She knew that this was a perfect choice, as she understood the hardships of being polar, not to mention of being blue. And she decided that she would give her special blessing to all polars, be they uni-, bi-, or as-yet-unaware-of-being- polar. Blue Joy knew she was going to have an extremely busy and productive blessing season.

The second question she faced was, "What special blessing should I bestow on all these myriad blue polars? An ice-making machine? No. Too cold. An electric blanket? No. Not exciting enough. How about blue hair? No. Too exciting." It became clear to Blue Joy that none of these things was, in the strictest invisibly significant sense, a true blessing.

70

After great thought, Blue Joy decided to consult Mom. Although Mom wasn't a blue polar, she understood everything and everybody and would know what blessing would be special, appropriate, and meaningful.

"Darling," said Mom, as affectionately as ever, "Blue polars don't really have an easy time of it, as you know perfectly well. How about giving them the love, respect, and understanding of all the other people in the world?"

Blue Joy was visibly disappointed. "But, Mom, that means I have to give those attributes to all the other people in the world, not to the blue polars. What sort of special blessing is that for the blue polars?"

"About the best I could ever imagine," replied Mom. And, of course, Mom, once again, was right.

And so Blue Joy in that very festive season blessed each and every person in the whole wide world who has a polar disorder with the love, respect, and understanding of all the other people in the whole wide world. She was absolutely thrilled to bestow this, her blessing of the millennium.

Try These Tactics

Those of us who experience recurring depressions have special responsibilities not shared by "normal" folk.

On top of the regular challenge of just getting by in the world, and growing, we must work out for ourselves how to manage painful and recurring episodes of the challenge that I like to call "mental unwellness."

I have, over the years, developed and implemented many strategies for keeping as healthy as I possibly can, in good times and in bad. In good times, it is not hard to work on several of these strategies. In bad times, I may only be able to take a stab at one of them. The important thing is to build them into my life as much as I am able at any time so they may give me even small reprieve and comfort when I am down. My strategies include:

Medication that works, prescribed by an expert

It's of little value to take a medication that doesn't have enough oomph to meet the symptoms of a mental disorder. Conversely, over-medication can rob a person of active participation in the world. Experimentation, under the supervision of a doctor, may be required until a workable medication and regimen are found.

I know the frustration of taking medication that is ineffective. Medical science is not perfect, but it is getting better, and we must persevere. It took me about 18 years to find a medication that works very well for my condition. If I hadn't come to this solution, I wouldn't be able to partake meaningfully in the following strategies.

Healthy relationships

Those of us with mood disorders require a support system of friends and family, even if we at times know we don't have much to give in return. One very good friend, or the support of a self-help group, may be all it takes.

Meaningful "work"

It is very difficult to concentrate when we are depressed, but doing a concrete activity (from a full-time job to a hobby) can bring us out of ourselves when we are low, if only for the time we actually do it.

Exercise

Walking is a very healthy, inexpensive, solitary or social activity that most of us can enjoy, even when feeling down. When we exercise the heart for even 20 minutes, our brains produce endorphins, which provide a release and relief from an unquiet mind. Fresh air is a tonic in itself.

Diet

Although it's very tempting to not eat in a healthy way during an episode, research has proven that too much sugar, though it tastes so good and pretends to be a satisfying substitute for good feelings, can worsen our state of mind. A good balanced diet is essential for good mental health.

Therapy

There are many useful therapies offered in the community. Some come with a price tag; others are provided by the medical system. Using professional services to get through an episode may shorten in time, or lessen in severity, the intense pain.

Spirituality

Belief that this episode will end is hard to find when one is unwell. Frequently the only light at the end of the cold, dark tunnel is the one that says "this too will pass." We must hold onto this promise.

Meditation

Meditation, prayer, reflection, and contemplation all lead us to a calmer state. The search for clarity and peace in our minds may not always be fruitful, but the act of seeking can in itself help generate a quiet within, and a momentary cessation of self-torturing thoughts.

Keeping well while we are feeling well helps us through down times. Although we may be unable to practice more than one of these strategies when we are low, a consistency of endeavor will help us. Each tiny moment of relief achieved through just one of the strategies is worth the effort.

The strategies come with no promises. And "strategy" does not imply "cure." Don't say to yourself: if I run or meditate or take pills, I will get better. The fact is that in time you will recover with or without these activities. Your illness has a mind and timetable of its own.

But each, or all, of these strategies, if practiced in your healthy life, will give relief, however small or brief, during the anguish of an episode.

Section 2:

Understanding and Refining

Visitors

Brent is a great downhill skier. Skiing has been his favourite sport since his Dad took him to the local hill when he was ten.

But skiing isn't the only downhill activity Brent takes part in. He has experienced depressive episodes (he likes to call them "my atrocious rides to hell") three times in his 21 years. He is a good actor when he has to be, thank heavens. Fortunately no one at school, not even the guys he hangs out with, has had any notion of his illness. Until recently, that is.

Brent hid his "mental affliction" (his own term for his mood disorder), from everyone except his family. Well, he could hardly hide it from Mom, could he? After all, she was the one who had taken him to see a psychiatrist after he'd had a real doozie of a downer in his last year of high school three years ago. He was damn sure to keep that from anyone outside the family.

On a college outing last winter, Brent broke his leg when he skied into an icy patch on a late afternoon run.

You stupid idiot, he scolded himself as he was being carried down the hill.

In the ambulance, in his drugged state, he imagined all his buddies visiting him at the hospital, giving him the gears for being such a klutz.

When the word got around campus that he had broken his leg, most of his friends did come to visit him.

Hey, I didn't realize I was so popular, he said to himself as four of his best pals left his room after a visit. *Sure is good to have close friends.*

A few months ago, Brent entered one of his downers. He immediately saw his psychiatrist, who told him to increase his anti-depressant medication.

Absolutely. It worked last time, so I should be fine in about three weeks.

But he wasn't fine in three weeks, or four weeks, or even five. He began to panic. His school work was suffering, and this was the final year of his program. As usual, when he had an episode, he kept mostly to himself, telling his friends he was studying hard. When he'd had an episode during the summer one year, he'd told his pals that he was sad and concerned about "a cousin who got ill suddenly."

Well, it was only a white lie, right? So it was my cousin's cousin. That's close enough, isn't it?

Things got worse. He sank lower than ever and was having thoughts about "doing something about this" (he couldn't use the word "suicide," though that's what he was thinking about), and his psychiatrist suggested that Brent go into hospital.

I must be really bad if he's suggesting that. But maybe it's a good idea for a day or two.

The psychiatrist arranged for Brent's admission, and Mom took him to the local hospital.

"The psychiatric ward is on Six West," the admitting clerk said automatically.

The psychiatric ward? Why should I be going to the psychiatric ward? I'm only depressed.

But he found out in no uncertain terms that the psych ward is where depressed patients landed up in this hospital.

Well, as long as my friends don't find out I'm here. I'll be out in a few days anyway, he assured himself.

But he wasn't out of the hospital in a few days. His best friend, Jim, had asked Brent's sister where he was. She wasn't comfortable with lying either, so she told him exactly where Brent was.

Oh well, I'll explain when he comes to visit that there weren't any beds in the other wards.

Two weeks passed, and no one had come to visit except his parents and his sister.

The guys probably thought I was going to be in here for only a couple of days, he concluded, remembering that he himself had thought that two weeks earlier.

Another two weeks passed, and Brent's depression was lifting slightly, but still no friends came to visit. He asked his sister whether anyone had asked after him.

"Oh, yes," she said. "But they don't understand your being in the hospital because you've never talked to them about your depression. They're all quite confused by it. By the way, I saw Jim today, and he asked me to say hi."

Four more weeks passed. He'd had no visitors except his family.

When the psychiatrist told him he'd improved enough to go home, he thought, *Well, the guys will certainly come to visit me now. They probably just don't like the feel of hospitals.*

A week passed at home. None of the guys visited, but Jim phoned and said, "It'll be great to see you back on campus."

Brent returned to school three months after he had plummeted. He was glad to be back, even though he would have to work hard to catch up on his school work. But he was still troubled that his friends hadn't visited him in the hospital or at home. He decided to ask a few of them about it.

He asked Jim first, because Jim had shown some interest. "I really thought you'd be out in a couple of days. It's sure good to have you back, man."

That's fair, Brent thought, *I'd thought the same myself.*

Then he asked Gary, who replied, "I've been pretty busy."

And Kevin, "I thought you wouldn't want to see anyone."

And Glenn, "To tell you the truth, I hate hospitals."

"But what about when I got home?"

"I was studying. I have a heavy course load this term."

He asked Lee, who responded, "I didn't know what to say."

"But you came to see me when I broke my leg. You could have said similar things, like 'How are you doing?' or 'The snow's lousy this year on the mountain.'"

"Yeah, well. Sorry I didn't."

Brent had heard enough reasons—no, they were excuses—from his friends. *I would have been satisfied to put up with any embarrassment in the hospital just to see my buddies.*

He decided to put it out of his mind. He couldn't afford to worry about it now, with exams coming up.

One day Jim stopped Brent in the corridor. He seemed nervous.

"Hey, guy. I need to talk to you."

"Sure." Brent was a bit cool.

81

"I'm really sorry I didn't visit you in the hospital, and then when you were at home... I didn't know what to say. I've never gone to visit anyone in the psych ward. You're my best buddy, and I let you down. I'm sorry." He paused.

"Thanks for saying that." Brent warmed up a bit.

"Well if there's ever a next time..." (Brent shivered at the thought.) "I'll definitely come to visit, if you'd like."

"I'd definitely like."

"Good. But I have a question."

"Shoot."

"Well, what... What should I say when I come by?"

Brent had had considerable time in the hospital and at home to think about what he would like to hear from his friends when he was ill.

"Oh, something like, 'Hi there, how's it going? Skiing's been crappy this year. Anything I can do for you?' Something like that."

"Really? Just regular stuff?"

"Really." Brent paused briefly.

"I know it's not easy to go to a psychiatric ward to visit. It wasn't much fun being there, I'll tell you. But it would be so good to see at least one of my buddies, to know that somebody realizes I'm not around. Or even to find out that I didn't miss any good skiing over the winter."

Jim relaxed noticeably. "You got it, pal. I promise. Shake on it?"

Brent and Jim shook hands. Boy, did it feel good.

I Don't Pretend Any More

I used to periodically pretend that I don't have a mood disorder. After all, experiencing depression over and over and over again is a very scary and painful reality. So why shouldn't I pretend I don't have it? If I pretend, and am successful at convincing myself, maybe, with a bit of luck, I can live like most other folks do.

This is a very dangerous mind game, and one I do not recommend.

A person in a wheelchair can never forget her dependence on that chair and on other people. Nor can a blind person pretend he is not blind, without dire consequences. But, with my "invisible impediment," I have at times, during stable periods, when my brain decides to behave itself, been very tempted to pretend and forget. So I have pretended.

How very lovely to see life as others do during these make-believe times, with "ordinary" ups and downs, being able to make plans and carry them through, having the confidence that a roulette wheel is not controlling my life. When I pretend, I obliterate large dismal chunks of my life and forget that I have spent all that valuable lifetime feeling poisonous, ugly, unacceptable, and unproductive.

I enjoy the wonderful fantasy for a while. Then, if I'm lucky, I return to my reality without negative consequence. Or, I may get caught.

When I am well, I live my life as others do, although I suspect I may be a bit more thankful for each healthy day that I'm given. When I am well, often the only reminder of my disorder is the fact that I take pills twice a day. When I am well, I don't constantly worry about or fear the time when I might experience another down episode. This absence of fear at times surprises me. So far in my life there has always been a next time.

Why don't I quiver and shake in fear? Because it would simply do no good, and life is too short.

When I'm well, I monitor my mood briefly each day, to sense whether I might be starting a downturn. If I didn't do this, I could be caught unawares, miss the early warnings, the subtle signs, and suddenly find myself on the slippery slope. Once I am on that slope, it's hard to stop. It's better to heed the early warnings, to take precautions (generally more medication, in my case), and possibly avoid the slide.

But sometimes, even when I monitor well and catch myself early, I cannot avoid the deep dark pit, with its ominous presence. At these times, I often try to deny that this is really happening. I'm loath to accept and admit that, "Yes, we're going to hell for a while," for, in that acknowledgment, I seem to be sentencing and propelling myself to that horrific place. But I shouldn't frantically try to escape the torment. That often only worsens it.

At the beginning of an episode, I'm very angry that I have this disorder. This anger is, in itself, healthy. But there's no point in lashing out at the world. The world has very little to do with this. I'm dealing here with brain chemistry. The only link anyone else has to my disorder is genetic. This illness has traveled faithfully through my family for several generations.

What I'm trying to do through this writing is to accept this disorder, as hard as that is, and to have compassion for myself. Knowing that I am entering a phase of bleak isolation, exhaustion, and depression is not easy. However, with acceptance of the cycles, I am easier on myself; I tend to blame myself less. With compassion, I know that what I have to do is wait, to not cry over lost time, and to continuously try to let go of self-deprecating thoughts.

It's extraordinarily difficult to accept these terrible interruptions in my life, but I don't know any other route to take. Yet.

Fish God

Susan always chooses Christmas presents very carefully for Linda. They have exchanged festive gifts for almost all of their lives, even now when they are living thousands of miles apart.

Susan always likes to get her friend something appropriate for whatever "season" Linda is in. She compares Linda's cycles of wellness to unwellness to wellness again to the seasons. She doesn't like to use terms like "uni polar mood disorder" and "episode." *They sound so clinical.*

Linda accepts whatever way Susan sees her illness, as long as she stands by her, which she always does.

This Christmas, Linda is in the recovering phase of an episode.

Sure has been a long spell, Susan sympathized.

She couldn't remember any other Christmas when Linda was coming out of a downer. Not that she could pinpoint anyway. Sometimes it's difficult to tell when Linda is recovering because it's such a jerky, erratic time, one day up, the next down.

How discouraging it must be some days, but now it really is the "springtime" of Linda's cycle.

Spring means new growth and gardening. Ah, yes. Gardening. Working with the earth has helped her get through more than one down. I'll give her something special for her garden this year!

Susan went to her favourite gardening store and looked around for that something special. She passed by the collection of rocks with inspirational sayings on them that everyone is buying these days: "Love," and "Joy," and "Dreams," etc.

Too trite.

She perused the collection of gardening books, plant holders, T-shirts, and ornaments.

She's got enough of those.

As she was leaving the shop without a gift, one of the rocks caught her eye. It had "Carpe Diem" carved on it.

Mmm... "Seize the Day." That's appropriate for Linda these days. It may help her through the rough patches while she's getting better.

It was a tough decision to make. Would it be helpful, but not pushy? On her more positive days, Linda would probably find it inspirational, but it may be too forceful when she has a vulnerable day.

Would she feel guilty or inadequate because she couldn't seize the day on a bad one? Well, she can always turn it over on the bad days.

She bought the rock, wrapped it, paid the considerable postage, and sent it off to Linda.

* * *

Although her recoveries are always unpredictable, Linda tries to be hopeful, but not unrealistically expectant, during this stage. Her slogan for these times is, "Take each day as it comes," and she's been reminding herself of that for weeks now.

On Christmas day, which she always spends with her family, Linda looks wistfully at the wrapped gift and imagines being with Susan. She feels sad because they aren't together, but also joy and comfort in knowing that she has such a faithful friend.

This is as heavy as a rock, Linda chuckles. She shakes it; there's no clinking. *Perfect. Something solid is exactly what I need these days.*

When she gets the wrapping off, she exclaims, "Oh, my God, it is a rock! What a strange gift. I wonder what I'm supposed to do with it."

"Carpe Diem."

Carpe Diem? Linda's Latin isn't too good, but she knows whatever it means will be perfect for her, because Susan always gives her perfect gifts.

She tries to guess what Carpe Diem means.

Carpe is a type of fish, I think. Diem? That sounds something like Deity, which I know means God. Mmm... Fish God? Could that be it? It's kind of bizarre. No, it can't be. Susan's never that obscure.

She thinks about it a bit longer, then gives in. Today she is able to go along with a game for a few minutes, but not any longer.

86

She knows that if she tries to guess much longer, she'll start to get agitated, maybe even angry, and that would take away from the spirit of the gift.

Stop guessing. Just look it up in the dictionary.

The dictionary tells her that Carpe Diem literally translates as, "Seize the day," which in plain English means, "Take each day as it comes."

I might have known. Susan's done it again. Another perfect gift.

She holds the rock in her hand, tracing the inscription with her fingers.

And if that saying ever bugs me on a down day, all I have to do is turn it over, but I bet Susan figured out that one, too!

Hide and Go Seek

It is very difficult and often impossible to recognize, not to mention diagnose and treat mental illness in its earliest stages. Many years of intense pain and confusion may pass before anyone recognizes that something is seriously wrong.

I hid my mood disorder, my terrible secret, for eight years, until I was suicidal. I see that long process of hiding and finally being found as similar to the popular children's game of hide-and-go-seek.

"Hide..."

I couldn't and wouldn't reveal my inner hell until the pain became unbearable. My inner obstacles to any intervention were:

- I was ignorant. I didn't know what was wrong in me. Was I "nuts"?
- I was afraid. My imagination convinced me that I had "cancer of the mind," which carried, I assumed, an automatic and early death sentence.
- I was intensely ashamed. I felt that I was a poisonous, useless, rotten girl. I felt guilt because I couldn't keep myself relatively happy like everyone else could.
- So, I became isolated. I was alone with my torment. No one knew I was hiding or in deep pain. No one could seek me out, and help me.

"...and go seek"

The responsibility of intervention in mental illness does not rest entirely with the afflicted, but also with the family, the school system, society in general, and the medical profession. They weren't much help to me 30 years ago.

Family obstacles

The lack of understanding about mental illness existed in my family. When I was in so much pain that I couldn't hide my darkness, my mother would say, "You'll feel better, dear. This just goes with being a teenager."

When my father finally recognized that my periodic withdrawal and bleakness were similar to those he had faced silently for years, he sent me to a psychiatrist. At that time psychiatrists had a reputation of treating only "loonies," so I didn't say a word to him.

My parents coveted the apparent good health of their offspring, so my treatment was very hush-hush; I was, unfortunately, the victim of their pride. Or was it shame?

School system obstacles

My school environment didn't provide me with any relief either. Teachers were uninformed about mental illness. They saw my problem as shyness. They assumed everyone could pull themselves up. After all, "we all get the blues now and then."

Other students were of no help. They couldn't be. The "loonie" label loomed large in my mind, so I didn't share my agony with any of my friends..

Commonly held beliefs

In the 1950s and 60s, the primary treatment for depressed individuals consisted of talking to a psychiatrist, and to mine I was faithfully silent. The only "options for treatment" to be had were in a psychiatric ward of a hospital, or, worse yet, in a psychiatric hospital. My youthful understanding of these places was that they were dreadful, and once in, you never got out. In addition, the word around town was that those "shrinks" were administering electric shock therapy to "almost everybody." I dug even deeper into my pit.

Medical system limitations

The medical profession itself was not able to cope successfully with mental illness when I first needed help. Research was underway but progressed slowly, and information and knowledge were sadly limited. Because my difficulty was deemed "depressed due to age or circumstance," my problem "obviously" couldn't be treated with medication.

"You're it"

Early intervention in mental illness is a "you and me" affair, requiring the compassion and awareness of many people. There are fewer external obstacles now than before. My family and friends have gained a good understanding of the illness and recognize its symptoms, and they encourage me to react sooner to a downturn. Public perception is not quite so harsh or misinformed, and medical knowledge has advanced.

"I'm it"

Intervention is not a one time act, but an ongoing need. My disorder manifests approximately once every three or four years, and each episode presents obstacles to, and opportunities for, early intervention. My inner obstacle today is an understandable resistance to a trip to hell. My personal responsibility is to take measures to minimize the stay.

One of these days hide-and-go-seek will be only a game.

Downward Bound

Liam knows that having one of those feeling low days doesn't necessarily mean that an episode of depression is imminent.

Having several bad days in a row, especially when he can't attribute his feelings to an external event such as a loss or a disappointment of some sort, means it is time to look at whether he may be experiencing symptoms of an episode.

After a few more days, he gets that sinking feeling. *This may be an episode.*

It's too soon, he moans.

He knows, of course, that any time is too soon, but this time it seems to be particularly soon. He takes a deep breath, knowing he mustn't panic.

I've got to carefully rule out any other possible reason for feeling low.

He goes through his usual personal diagnostic checklist.

- Could it be the weather?
  No, it's been sunny for two weeks, and I've been soaking it up. Besides, weather never seems to trigger an episode for me. Best to check though, just in case."
- Have I experienced a trauma of late?
  No, I've just been living life quite ordinarily. My parents are in good health. Ashley and I are doing fine. I quit smoking 3 years ago, so it can't be withdrawal.
- Am I worried or fearful about anything?
  Nothing I can think of, except another episode.
- Am I going through any major changes right now?
  No, I moved a year ago, and I'm happy with my new digs. Everything else is stable too, as far as I'm concerned.

Liam's mood slips even more in the next few days. He has exhausted all rational explanations for feeling depressed. He decides it's time to tell his Mom, Ashley, and his best friend, Jason, about his state of mind. He didn't tell them sooner because he didn't want them to worry. After all, it could still be only a "blip." As usual, they are sympathetic, supportive.

Thank heavens for that. Some people don't get that backup.

He calls his doctor, who tells him to increase his morning medication by one capsule, "and don't forget you won't get the benefits of it for six weeks or so," he cautions, adding insult to injury.

Well, that makes it absolutely official. It's the pits for me again. Damn!

As he expects, after a couple of days Liam is physically exhausted. And then his intellect goes to pot.

It's three out of three this time obviously.

Yes, this time he's been hit by the "Thieving Three": debilitating mood, exhaustion, and mental chaos.

Now he must determine what other decisions he needs to make. He's self-employed and happens to not be working on a contract at the moment, which is a blessing. He decides to carry on with the camera club for the time being.

I need an outlet, something to get me out of the house at least once a week, even though it's tough to face those people when I'm depressed.

Then he gets out the "Daily List for When I'm Sick," his guide to get him through each painful day.

Going down happens quickly this time. The rapid descent means dramatic changes, which he can see, so he can make necessary adjustments early on.

With his previous episode, he was unaware of his diminishing capabilities because they happened so slowly. His work suffered, and he was almost fired. He knew people were looking at him skeptically. After that mess, he asked Jason and Ashley and his mother to tell him when they noticed any changes, however minor, in his behavior, so he could adjust accordingly.

At least I haven't embarrassed myself this time.

Over the next few days, Liam makes some silly mistakes. Instead of taking library books back to the library, he takes some of his own books. He becomes increasingly confused and forgetful. After embarrassing himself a couple of times, he decides to withdraw from contact with other people.

It's not worth the humiliation. I feel so ashamed of having this dumb illness.

94

He gets a flashback to earlier horrible down times. He panics, and his panic leads to anger.

This isn't fair. I just came out of a bloody episode, for heaven's sake. I hate feeling totally isolated like I am now.

He wants to give up, admit defeat. He used to throw his arms up and cry something like, "I may as well give in to this monster!" But he knows better now. He knows, too, that fighting is not going to get him out of this mess and that fleeing is not an option. The only sensible response to the painful situation is acceptance.

How many years has it taken me to realize that?

Accepting this hell is, of course, almost impossible to do. But Liam makes the immense effort.

Again, damn it!

As usual, his acceptance is clouded by understandable bitterness.

He experiences the usual consequences that his illness and self-isolation bring. Now those nasty fears appear: that he won't be able to get work when he gets better, that he might harm himself, that his girlfriend may want to break up with him.

I always worry about that, but she's hung in all this time.

But that doesn't make him feel any better, any more secure.

The fears multiply and collide in Liam's closed mind. They are so intense that he starts to fear the worst things.

Maybe I'm going mad. Maybe this is a psychosis. Yes, it probably is. But why hasn't my shrink figured it out yet?

So many maybes. He's afraid to bring them up with anyone, even his psychiatrist. His fear turns to torment, his torment to dread.

This is going to last forever; I can tell. He knows he is on a steep slippery slope, and has no control. *This downer is going to be deadly.*

No. No, I don't really mean "deadly."

Liam has never had suicidal thoughts. He's not sure why, but he's immensely grateful for small mercies.

He knows there's going to be darkness, despair, and a lot of desolation. And now it's a matter of waiting. Waiting for almost forever.

If he has learned anything from too many past episodes, it is to wait patiently for them to end. Now he gets to practice again, waiting for who knows how long.

What else can I do, anyway?

Approaches

A group of 30 people from all walks of life with mood disorders of various sorts volunteered to answer a one-question survey. The question was, "What approach will you take when you recognize you are entering your next depressive episode?" Here are several of their responses.

I'll hold on for dear life until it's over. Otherwise I may not come out of it, ever.

I'll flush my stupid pills down the toilet, for all the good they do me. Then I'll panic and phone my doctor for more.

All I have to do is grit my teeth, put on shoulder pads, and plow my way through it. What works on the football field works in life, our coach said. Sounds good to me.

I'll feel sorry for myself, as usual. Poor me, again.

I'll start taking my medication again. The way I see it I don't need pills when I'm feeling well, and being productive. I don't know if they really make any difference when I'm down, but I resent having to spend money on pills when I'm healthy.

I'll just give into it again—the self-hate and torment. Another episode is inevitable. I've had downs faithfully for the past 35 years, every winter. No matter what I do, they come back with the same vengeance. I just wait until it's over, then try to crawl out of the pit again, usually in about March. As they say: if you can't beat it, join it.

I'll hate myself. I always do.

I don't know. I don't want to think about it. It could start another downward slide.

It depends. If my next downer is mostly an energy problem, I'll cut back on my activities. If it hits my mood mostly, I'll try not to berate myself, and meditate daily. Those things have worked before for me.

I'm never going to get depressed again. Period. I can't afford to, with the children still so young. Besides, I'm feeling so well now I'm sure I'll never feel that sick again. I <u>won't</u>! It's mind over matter.

I'm going to "ride" it until I'm through it, try to accept that it is with me again. I've learned a few things in my 42 years: get lots of rest, reduce stress, be kind to myself (as much as I can under the circumstances). These things help but cannot obliterate the Ominous Beast. I've found that out over the years.

You tell me. I'm no good at it.

I'LL GO INTO HIDING. I CAN'T STAND PEOPLE SEEING WHAT AN AWFUL PERSON I AM WHEN I'M DOWN. I FEEL TOO ASHAMED AND GUILTY TO SHOW MY FACE.

First I'll pretend it's not here, then I'll SCREAM, then I'll have a huge fight with my partner, then I'll feel guilty, then I'll be remorseful, then I'll be morose. Then, probably, it will be over and I'll have another high.

I'll just eat and sleep. Who cares anyway?

I'll feel so crummy. I usually take sick leave from my job— never see anyone. I feel horribly alone, but I don't have any choice, do I?

I'll beat the sucker. I read about this great, new technique in that **Cure Yourself of Depression Forever** book they're all talking about these days. All you have to do is... No, you'll have to read it for yourself. But trust me, it's simple and brilliant. For the first time in my life I'm ready for my next downer.

I'll start smoking again. That will teach it something.

Reading Rules

Robin has learned a thing or two as a result of the four episodes he has had to date. He thinks he is a painfully slow learner at times.

But it's bloody hard living with this stupid illness, he tells himself.

Each episode is unique and challenges him in different ways. Each episode has so many setbacks, and disappointments. And each episode has opportunities for learning.

Take, for instance, this current episode. As usual, Robin is choosing to do lots of reading, his favourite pastime. Nothing, as far as he is concerned, is more interesting, inspiring, or motivating than reading, reading, and more reading, at the best and the worst of times.

He learned a few years back that when he is feeling isolated and extremely vulnerable, going to the library and being in the company of other folks (but not having to interact with them) made him feel safer. He was so relieved when he discovered this strategy, this safety valve.

Last week he went to the library and picked up a book. The only problem was that he picked up just any old book. Then he forced himself to read it completely in one sitting. He thought it might get his mind off feeling so lousy, but instead, his mind spun right out. After about an hour, it felt like the library closed in on him. He lost track of where he was, what day it was, almost who he was. This was terribly frightening to Robin, who already felt pretty awful.

So, he decided it was time to develop some reading rules. This may sound strange, but it was absolutely necessary, for otherwise, he wouldn't be able to read at all during his episodes, which was unthinkable.

Here is the first of Robin's **Reading Rules**:

> **If you can't concentrate on reading a book, magazine, _anything_, STOP READING IT.** Put the book down; stand up and walk around.

More rules quickly came to mind.

When he is down, Robin likes to read kids' books, but he has felt foolish doing so. He realized that it was foolish to feel foolish. So he made this rule:

> **Reading a kid's books is absolutely fine.** Hiding a kid's book inside an adult book is okay.

As he made up each new rule, Robin wrote it in a very "Do this" manner, as if someone else was instructing him, so that the rules would have a strong impact when he was in difficulty. They would be imperatives, and he would be more likely to follow them.

Another rule he made up that day, based on a long history of bad experiences, was:

> **Don't force yourself to read anything in particular.**
>
> Even if everyone says, "This is the greatest book going."
>
> It may not be a good one for you *now*. Jot down the title for a healthier time.

Three good rules, he told himself proudly.

He resolved to take his Rules along every time he went to the library. He knew he had a tendency to forget important things when he was depressed.

One day, Robin picked up a new book, "Life in the Perilous Pit" (fictitious title). He sat down in a cubicle and began reading it. Actually, he tried to devour it. The first chapter frustrated him because his mind wasn't concentrating. He couldn't remember a word of the second chapter. He kept reading, oblivious to his first rule. By page 50, he was more in the dumps than he had been at any time during the entire episode.

Then he remembered his Reading Rules.

Time to add some new rules, he decided.

Due to his muddled head, and general bad mood, it took him a very long time to figure out what that new rules should be. Eventually he came up with two new rules.

> Glance at a new book when you pick it. up—don't let it consume you.

> Keep your reading stints short and look at your watch or a clock frequently to make sure.

It's always important to let the message go deep at the time I create it, he reminded himself, *even if I forget it when I need it!*

After reading these new rules about 10 times, Robin thought he had really absorbed them.

On his way home, Robin thought, *Hey, I'm doing really well making up rules when I'm depressed. Maybe I could think of even more rules when I'm in good health. I think I'll have a go at that when I've recovered. Better make a note of that in case I forget.*

Something to learn every day, he sighed.

Choosing Words Wisely

Life is tough enough for those of us who experience recurring depressions. We don't need to complicate it further by communicating poorly with someone who shows an interest in how we are doing.

If you're like me when I'm in the depths of an episode, you don't feel like saying much of anything to anybody. Truth be known, our feelings at that time may be, "I'm angry that I'm feeling absolutely rotten. I hate this place, and I don't want to talk about it." Fortunately, I'm usually able to hold myself back from saying that.

It's neither fair nor wise to take out our mental pain on someone else. A rude response does injustice to both parties. A rude or curt remark could confuse, offend, or hurt a compassionate friend or family member, and we'd all end up feeling worse.

Are there any ways to respond differently, and better? Certainly there are. An appropriate response may be different each time we're asked about our state of health. It depends on how "out" about our illness we are with the questioner, and how vulnerable we feel at the time. It is perfectly okay to be vague sometimes, and sometimes it is absolutely necessary. But it's not a good idea to leave someone with more questions than answers.

Let's look at a few scenarios.

* * *

A concerned acquaintance asked Sally, "Is something bothering you? You seem a bit distant." Because she was feeling absolutely dreadful, Sally responded, "I'm depressed all the time, and I can't do anything about it."

That's not much of an invitation to the comfort and support that her friend could offer. Besides, was she really depressed "all the time?" It does seem like that when we feel utterly horrible, but that statement would sometimes be stretching the truth a bit.

Sally could have better responded with, "Sorry I seem that way. I don't mean to. It's just that I really am feeling out of sorts these days."

* * *

Brad doesn't say much when he's in an episode because it takes so much energy to talk. So, when someone comments sympathetically, "You look stressed," he often opts for "Oh, well," leaving the other person with nothing more to say.

Brad might instead have responded with the more meaningful, "Well, I'm feeling quite low these days, and it's pretty exhausting."

* * *

Sometimes it may be too big a risk, or would in fact be unwise, to be totally honest about our illness. To allay possible nervousness or embarrassment, it's good to be prepared with a fitting response to a general question or comment in case you're presented with one.

For instance, if you don't want to be open with Todd, and he says, "You're looking blue," you might just say, "Yes, I am feeling a bit under the weather." If he asks, "Anything I can do?" You could respond, "I don't think so. But thanks for asking anyway."

* * *

How we respond to someone's interest, if we don't think it out properly, can really backfire on us.

For instance, if Jen commented to her workmate, Pat, "You don't look very happy," and Pat responded, "Oh, I'm just wiped." The fact may be that Pat is most depressed at that time of day and is frightened of being alone.

But Jen might think "Pat's obviously not feeling well. Sounds like she wants to be by herself. Guess I'd better just leave."

It would have been better, for her own sake, if Pat had said something like, "I'm feeling depressed these days, and this is my toughest time of day. I know I'm not great company right now, but I do appreciate that you're here with me."

* * *

We often have a choice of responses to questions and comments about our well-being. We can often make a meaningful and fitting choice before being forced by a situation to react to someone's interest. If we think ahead, we may experience less stress when we are depressed, and *that* is a good thing.

Word Game

Craig prides himself on being a word person—that is, when he is feeling well, which she definitely wasn't, as he stared blankly at his computer screen.

It stared back at him, absolutely black, just like him. The only interruption on the screen was "This too will pass," scrolling from right to left very slowly across the silent bleakness.

Sure, he sighed to himself. *"This" as in this day, this hour, or this minute?* he asked no one; though he knew perfectly well that "This too" meant his current episode of depression.

Episode, he pondered. *Episode. They should call this bloody interference in my life a "trip to hell," or, to placate Mom, a "trip to heck."*

But even that hardly expressed the state he was in. He could come up with lots of really bad words to define his mood, but the rules didn't allow that.

His mother had reminded him at lunch that, "Today's the day, you know." In a weak moment Craig had made a deal with her that he would change the message on his computer screen each week, come heck or high water. So, that became the first rule. It was about the only thing he could agree to, or carry out, these days.

Mind your own business, Craig thought.

"Yeah Mom, I know," he said. He didn't mind Mom making the odd suggestion when he was in the pits, as long as she didn't follow up her grand ideas with "It may help," or "Do it, son." He couldn't stand people telling him what to do when he was down, even though he couldn't figure out for himself what to do next.

But she was right, which is why he was staring at the monitor.

I never knew black could be so deep, he thought, and morosely chuckled.

He couldn't think of anything with which to replace that stupid "This too..." statement from last week. He'd only thought of that phrase because some dork had said it to him recently.

What else have people said? He dug as deeply into his fuzzy brain as he could, which was about half an inch.

Why do there always have to be rules? he asked himself, then remembered that he had made up all the rules himself. He didn't need rules when he was well, because he was a word person, and word persons can find things to say. Except when they are depressed.

Another rule was that he had to change the background colour of the screen each week. Mom had said, "Well, dear, black is dramatic," when he had chosen last week's colour. She wasn't too bad a sort, really. She knew where to stay when he was ill—not too close, not too distant.

So, Craig could not just leave the screen black.

How about dark purple? Or a dirty forest green, or navy with a hint of red representing the life seeping out of me?

No, he couldn't do that, because another rule was that if he had a dark colour one week, it had to be a light colour the next.

Damn, why did I do this to myself? he berated himself, which was so easy to do these days.

He reluctantly chose orange, usually his favourite colour, but at these times black was the only colour, if you could call it one, that appealed to him. Colour-change done, now all he had to do was choose a saying, a slogan, a phrase. A rule about that was it had to be non-negative.

That means it doesn't have to be positive, thank heavens. It can be neutral.

That was the best he could do at these times anyway.

All he had to do.... He hated it when people said, "All you have to do...." His teacher had counseled, "All you have to do is be kind to yourself." His dumb sister had offered, "All you have to do is look on the bright side."

All you have to do is climb Mount Everest when you're depressed and then you'll get better, he had wanted to reply each time.

But that would only make people feel sorry for him, and he couldn't stand that. So he remained mute, which was his most common condition when he was depressed.

His final rule, which was the toughest, was that the saying had to have meaning to him right this minute. He couldn't write, for instance, "I am a great guy," because that was a lie these days as far as he was concerned. Besides, he was the one who had to look at the message on the screen, and he didn't want to throw up all the time.

One new word in Craig's vast vocabulary *(hardly vast right now,* he snickered) was "labile" meaning liable to change, unstable.

Yes, well, that's exactly me these days. He congratulated himself on being able to say that this word had meaning to him right this minute.

And it's not negative, really, he continued. He was getting quite excited at the prospect of using his new word on the orange screen. *This is a pretty stupid thing to get excited about,* he thought, but, being a word person, he was allowed.

He sat in front of his blank orange screen for about an hour, trying to work out a suitable saying with "labile" in it.

It doesn't really rhyme with anything, he lamented. *Actually, it's a pretty ridiculous word.*

He could almost hear his English teacher saying, "Now, Craig, a person with your ability should be able to work that word into a sentence."

Aha! That was it. He had his statement! It was non-negative, it meant something to him now, and it went well with orange!

Quickly, before he could talk himself out of it, he typed it in: "Lability will be replaced eventually by ability"

Who cares if "lability" is or isn't a word? There's no rule about that.

Craig felt great. He had done something today. He was able to think.

Well, sort of, if you could call that thinking.

Craig got up from his chair and watched his scrolling brilliance for a few minutes. He left his room and promptly plunged back into his darkness.

At least I had that moment, he sighed as he crashed.

Deal with It

I had been completely out of my most recent episode for about four months. It had been no worse than other episodes. In fact, it had been better, if one can use the word better for something that is essentially hell. Anyway, it was over. I was swimming and socializing once again, and looking forward to my plans for the winter.

The episode had been characterized mostly by physical exhaustion. During the worst months, my mood was bleak and I was quite confused, but it was lack of energy that plagued me most. It hung on me like a wet blanket for three months after the other symptoms had subsided.

I had promised myself many times during this foggy period, *When this is over, I'm going to find a new medication that will prevent me from becoming so worn out.*

Being tired for the better part of every day for three months after my mood had improved, was discouraging, to say the least. I could think clearly, but without the physical horsepower I was unable to do anything of any value or duration.

But I was able to dream about taking only one medication instead of the cocktail that I'd been on for five years.

I made an appointment to see a psychiatrist who specializes in medication for mood disorders. I told him that I was taking three medications. I told him the dosage of each. And I told him that I was sick and tired of so many pills.

I told him that a friend of mine from a support group was now on one medication, a new one combining the virtues of two older ones, and another friend had been able to cut back to two from four.

Three pills in one would be great, thanks, was the request I was leading up to.

After listening to me for about 10 minutes, he looked straight at me and asked, "You think that one medication will do you now?"

"Yes." was my eager reply.

"Well, I'm afraid it's not so simple in your case."

In my case. In my case? What's so different about my case?

111

"I divide people with recurring depression into three groups," the psychiatrist continued, as if he'd heard my question. "The first group can be treated successfully with one medication. It may change over time, but one is sufficient to combat their symptoms." He waited for a moment.

"The second group can be treated successfully with two medications, usually, though not always, an anti-depressant and a mood stabilizer." He paused.

"The third group, your group, has to be treated with more than two medications. The fact of the matter is that no two medications available today are sufficient to alleviate the severe symptoms of your illness."

Severe symptoms? Don't other people have symptoms as bad as mine? Am I that different, that much worse than others who experience episodes of depression?

"What do you mean?" I asked, trying to appear calm.

"Well, you have a very serious mood disorder, and extraordinary measures are necessary to deal with it."

And here I'd been thinking, hoping, that a new medication, one magic pill, would solve my physical exhaustion along with everything else.

"But I hate having to take so many pills. I'm so embarrassed that I don't tell anyone how much I'm taking. They'd think that I was really sick. I thought with all the recent advances and the success stories I've read about, that things would get easier for me." I was very upset.

The psychiatrist responded quietly, "The fact is that you would probably have an absolutely horrendous episode if you didn't take the medications you do."

This was very difficult for me to listen to. I knew full well how awful my episodes were, but I'd concluded that they were that way just because I wasn't adept at going through them gracefully.

"I don't like being held captive by so many medications," I said weakly.

"Well, deal with it," he replied, looking me straight in the eye.

Deal with it. DEAL WITH IT? My mind raced trying to find a way out of this corner. I didn't want to deal with anything. I just wanted one pill to fix everything.

I went home feeling dejected. I'd have to continue to be vague if people asked about my medication. I realized that I had a more serious illness than I had ever thought, and that I'd have to be more careful about taking extra medication with me whenever I went anywhere.

A few weeks later, when I'd settled down with the psychiatrist's news and thought about it sensibly, I decided I was better off knowing the magnitude of my illness. I could feel less guilty that my episodes are so terrible, so frequent, and so lengthy. I could release myself from the lies I'd been feeding myself. The truth may have hurt, but it could also lighten the load I had put on myself.

I like to think that someday research will be able to offer me a single anti-depressant that will work better than the three I need now. But until then I must, I can and I will accept today's necessity.

Table for Two

Day 74. Carrie knows it's Day 74 because she marks the days off in groups of five (卌). She uses the blackboard because in her current state she can't keep track of a single piece of paper. This has been her ritual since she first started having these dreadful episodes. It's been 74, long, horrid days so far this time.

Carrie is a gregarious person when she is well, but keeps to herself when she is ill. It's too hard—no, it's impossible—for her to concentrate on conversation or any ongoing activity when she is ill. What she does, essentially, is just wait, in silence and alone, until the episode is over. (She has come, over time, to think of an episode as a painful, impossibly long period of holding her breath.)

Whenever she's ill, Carrie goes to weekly support group meetings. This is about the only commitment she can keep during these times; though if her companion Leslie doesn't phone to remind her to go, Carrie herself certainly won't remember.

Each week when it's her turn to say something to the group, she tells them how many days she has been in this episode. That's it. Nothing more. No one else seems to keep track of how long their episodes last, or how many weeks or months it has been since their last one. But each week she offers her number of days. Period.

Leslie has tried, during Carrie's last two episodes, to get her friend to say more to the group, but she hasn't been successful. Other group members tell how they coped over the past week, whether they'd told anyone new about their disorder, what new strategies have helped them cope. That sort of thing.

Supporters often ask other supporters how they cope with particular situations, and members now in good health offer suggestions that might be helpful.

At one meeting, Raymond said to Daniel, who was desperately low, "It will pass; it always does." That was pretty hard for Daniel to stomach at the time, but they were words of hope nonetheless. And, of course, he did get better eventually.

Believing that Carrie could benefit from sharing some of her painful experiences with the group, Leslie decided to bribe her.

115

"I'll take you out to lunch if you say something next week about what's helping you get through this episode, and 'This is day whatever' doesn't count."

Carrie was not enthusiastic. "I've no idea what to say."

"You have a whole week to figure it out."

"Okay, if it'll get you off my case, I'll try."

And anyway, she thought, *one of the few things I enjoy doing when I'm sick is going out for a meal, and Leslie doesn't seem to mind the silence.*

Day 75. As usual, Carrie went to a coffee house near her home. In this quiet place, she always feels safe and anonymous. What a relief that is. Every day she orders a large latté and bran muffin. Having constants in her daily life is important to her these days.

Carrie always sits at a table that seems to her to be suitable for one person, though all the tables have a second chair. On her first visit, Carrie considered removing the chair (*just in case someone gets the idea to sit with me*) but realized that doing so would be a bit extreme. Someone might wonder.

Each day, Carrie sits for an hour or so, sipping her latté, writing in her journal, gazing out the window, and once in a while noticing the pleasant classical music in the background.

"Excuse me."

Carrie was snapped out of her fuzzy reflection by a male voice. She looked up.

"Is this seat taken?"

Carrie looked around. All the tables were occupied; in fact there were only two empty chairs in the café.

"Uh, well, no, no it isn't," she said, but thought, *I don't like it when I'm interrupted.*

So, whoever-this-was sat down. Carrie pulled her journal closer. It was a knee-jerk reaction, but hardly necessary. No one could read her writing at the best of times right side up, let alone her depressive scribbles upside down.

"Pretty nasty weather these days," he said in a friendly manner.

Oh, hell. Now my morning is ruined.

"Sure is." She hoped a short reply would discourage any further conversation.

"Writing a novel?"

Carrie tried to send a telepathic message. *Look at my face, mister, and you'll know I don't want to be disturbed.*

"No, just my journal," she replied vaguely.

"Hey, I do that too!"

Now she knew she was in the company of a very chatty person. *What a drag.*

Suddenly her blurry mind recalled Leslie's bribe. *If I talk to this guy I'll get my treat!*

She straightened up in her chair and tried to look more interested. Talking to him intelligently was going to be a major challenge.

What can I talk about? Certainly not about my illness. What have I been doing lately that could be of interest? Absolutely nothing. Oh, hell! I can't let him get away.

She dug further into her scrambled mind. She looked closely at him, wondering what his interests might be.

He looks sort of artsy. I don't have anything artsy to say. Oh, help!

"Number 26," a voice called out, and he went to pick up his order.

Out of the blue Carrie remembered a saying from her writing class. "Write about what you know best."

Yes! I should talk about what I know best. But all I know right now is that it's Day 75, and I'm depressed. I can't talk about that. I'd feel too exposed.

He sat down with his tea and toast, and then it came to her.

"Thanks for lunch," she said with a strong, clear voice. For the first time in weeks she felt a smile coming on.

"Pardon me?"

"I know it sounds weird, but because I'm talking to you now, I'm going to be treated to lunch by a friend."

He looked puzzled.

"What I mean is..." Carrie took a deep breath, and she told him about her depression, that she counts the days of each dreadful episode, and about Leslie's bribe.

Then she panicked.

Oh God. I've made an absolute fool of myself. Please God, let me disappear.

He interrupted her thoughts. "You know, I'm really glad you told me that."

"Really?"

"A good friend of mine has periods of depression—episodes as you call them. I've always wanted to know more about it, but I've been afraid to ask him. I'd like to help if I could, if I knew how. Would you... would you mind telling me more about it?"

You bet I wouldn't mind! I'm an expert on this topic. "I'd be pleased to."

Carrie felt as if a heavy load had lifted. She could actually offer something to another person when she's feeling horrible!

They talked for about half an hour. It was so good for both of them.

When they left the café, he felt wiser, and she felt doubly blessed for having helped him towards understanding, and for having lightened her load just by talking.

Don't Panic

You wake up. You're not feeling quite right. Perhaps you're gloomy, or exhausted, or can't remember what you're supposed to do even though you planned today's activities yesterday.

Things have been going along so smoothly for so long, you'd almost forgotten you ever get depressed. But this morning is different.

When you get to work, you're edgy and self-critical, and you want to avoid your colleagues.

What's going on? What do you do?

Your instinct may be to panic. *Oh, my God, I'm going into an episode!*

You ask yourself what you've done to deserve an episode now. Or you ask yourself what you should've done that you haven't.

If this is an episode, I've brought it on myself. It's all my fault.

You've fallen into the trap. You want to turn back the clock and start the day again, this time without the nightmare. Not possible.

How do you escape this mess? You try to calm yourself, but the memories of earlier down times gush into your mind and take over. You lose all perspective of where your life was going before this morning.

Whoa! Rather than panicking and sinking deeper into this mire, ask yourself some important questions.

Quiet questioning may help you determine whether this is an episode coming on, or not. Your answers may indicate what has precipitated this bad morning. Of course, there may not have been a precipitator; you may have just gotten out of bed on the wrong side. It's happened before. In any case, it's best not to immediately jump to the conclusion that your next episode is inescapably descending on you.

The act of questioning, the orderly process of asking and answering, is in itself therapeutic. It can help you to settle down for a bit and allow you to make more rational decisions about whatever it is you are facing.

Common reasons for normal depression:

Ask yourself...	**Why the question is relevant:**
Did you recently stop smoking, or try to give up some other habit?	Withdrawal from nicotine can have depressing effects, as can any abrupt change to your daily pattern.
Have you been exercising more than usual?	If you ask your body to do more than it's used to, you may be more tired than usual
Are you suffering from a recent painful injury or illness?	Pain can cause one to feel frustrated and dispirited.
Have you recently had, or do you have the flu, or other sickness?	Any illness that causes loss of energy can masquerade as depression.
For women: Could this be premenstrual syndrome (PMS), or are you going through menopause?	Some women feel low before their periods, and many women experience depression at some point during menopause.
Are you using over the counter medication (antihistimines, decongestants, Aspirin, Tylenol, etc.) as well as medication prescribed for depression?	Over the counter medication may interact badly with prescribed medication. Check with your doctor before using over the counter drugs.

Could be an episode, or not:

Ask yourself...	**Why the question is relevant:**
Has a traumatic event happened recently in your life? Have you lost your job? Has a loved one died recently?	Some people think that personal traumas can make one more vulnerable to an episode. In any case, they can make one feel despondent.
Have you had an argument with someone close to you?	A personal upset may seem to, but rarely does, precipitate an episode.
Have you just finished a job, or a term at school?	One can experience a let down after sustained or arduous activity.
Has your best friend recently left town? Have you recently moved? Are you anxiously awaiting important news?	Loneliness, upheaval, and anxiety cause many of us to feel somewhat depressed. But feeling low does not necessarily mean an episode is imminent.
Is a long weekend looming, and you hate long weekends? Is it December, and you have always dreaded Christmas?	Distress associated with a dreaded event may seem like a symptom of depression.
Has the weather been grey and rainy, or hot and sticky for the past month or so?	Many week of the same weather, be it good or bad, can get anyone down.

Do you have something difficult to do or decide that you don't want to face?

People can get sick to avoid things they fear or dread.
They don't get sick on purpose. It just happens. They may end up feeling gloomy and ill-tempered for some time.

Possible episode indicators:

Ask yourself...

Why the question is relevant:

Have you been taking the prescribed amount of your medication(s) in the past few days, weeks?

If you are taking less medication than you should, your body may not be getting what it needs.

Has your doctor increased or decreased the dosage of one of your medications in the past 6 weeks, or are you in the process of switching from one medication to another?

In the midst of changing types of dosages of medication, it is not uncommon for one to experience symptoms of depressive illness while the body adjusts.

Have you been keeping your medication(s) in a cool, dry place, out of sunlight?

Medications stored in warm, humid, bright places may not work as intended.

Do you think it is time for you to have an episode? Do you usually have episodes at regular intervals and now your time is up?

Some of us have episodes "like clockwork." But cycles may change. You may be spared for another month or year.

| Have you been diagnosed with Seasonal Affective Disorder (SAD), and winter is coming on? | People who have SAD are more vulnerable to an episode when there are fewer daylight hours. |

This list may raise additional questions for you, or give you an idea of why you feel low today. If possible, discuss your concern with someone who has seen you through at least one episode. He or she may be able to help pinpoint the cause or ease the fear.

If you are still unsure, phone your doctor and discuss your situation. Have your answers to the above questions at hand. Follow your doctor's instructions. Do not alter the amount of medication you take unless your doctor instructs you to do so.

Be aware of mood shifts over the next few days. Soon you will know whether or not this is going to be a real episode.

In Spite of Herself

She was exhausted. She was on the verge of crying. She knew her soul had died. Lisa was, in a word, depressed.

She stared at herself in the mirror, and she detested what she saw. To avoid any further pain and self-humiliation, she quickly shut her eyes and turned away.

"Get rid of this rubbish inside yourself right now." She started to rebuke herself cruelly again. But the denseness and darkness ran through her blood, fed her muscles until they were dead weights, and filled her heart with the all too familiar dreaded self-abhorrence.

Lisa tried. She tried and tried and tried to obliterate the loathsome perception she had of herself, along with every other horrible feeling and thought that surged through her mind. She had even thought of killing the Ominous Presence, the awful demon that ran her life at times like this. But she knew that killing it would mean killing herself, and she wasn't ready for that, yet.

The doctor had told her it would take three weeks or so for the anti-depressant to take effect again. Yes, again. Lisa admitted to herself that stupidly she had gone off her medication once more—all because she was feeling so good, and couldn't imagine ever getting depressed again. That was then (a short two weeks ago), and this is now. Now, she couldn't fathom what "feeling good" meant. In her current, horrendous state, they were just two meaningless words.

She always swore, at this painful bottom of the repeating cycle, that she would never cut back on her pills again when she was feeling well. But, almost every time she was in a healthy mental state, she couldn't relate to that promise, or to the atmosphere in which it was made. So almost every time, her promise went out the window. Time and time and time again.

Lisa asked herself, again, what it would take to not be that stupid idiot, again.

Maybe if I hurl enough rubbish at myself, I'll learn. Maybe if I don't increase my medication now, I'll suffer more, and learn from that. Maybe if I...

She was getting very sick and tired of maybe-ifs.

Her doctor had told her more than once of a support group for people who have depressions. No. She could deal with this on her own, thanks all the same.

But now she was desperate. There was a meeting coming up. She felt strangely compelled to go, to overrule the equally strong force warning her that, "it's just another pie-in-the-sky."

Lisa didn't know how she got to the meeting, except by putting one heavy foot in front of the other. She was so nervous, distressed, depressed, and fuzzy-minded that she could hardly remember her name when someone asked.

During the meeting, one person claimed that the kind of depression that people coming to these meetings have is physically based.

Oh, right, Lisa mumbled to herself, cynically. *What a load of bunk. Next they'll tell me that it isn't my fault.*

"Is that how you see it, Lisa?" The facilitator's voice broke her train of thought, and Lisa had no idea what the speaker, or the group, had been talking about.

"Uh, what was it again, please?" She hoped no one would realize she was a million miles away and also in this room—both, somehow, at the same time, for who knows how long.

"Ben said that he was able to accept his disorder only after he looked at it as being similar to diabetes. It's a bio-chemical imbalance in his brain, he says, and he knows he must take medication for the rest of his life to maintain a healthy balance in his brain."

This sounded like a lot of hogwash to Lisa, but she wasn't about to say that at her first meeting. "I've never thought of it that way," she replied safely.

She couldn't get out of that meeting fast enough when it ended. Thoughts were swirling in her head, testimonials that she desperately wanted to believe, but daren't. "It's not my fault." "I'm finally on the right medication." "My acceptance of my disorder as a physical problem has kept me healthy for eight years now." Hearsay, heresy, nonsense, all sense.

126

Lisa vowed she'd never go to one of those dumb meetings again, and then proceeded to dissect everything she had heard that evening.

Those people are just kidding themselves, she thought, against her own yearning. She didn't want to appear hopeful, even in front of herself. *But... What if...?*

She mulled it all over. Over and over and over.

Might there be something in what they said?

Maybe, just maybe, this disorder was not her fault, maybe she really did have faulty brain chemistry, and maybe the right medication could set her brain straight.

Eventually she decided to find out about it, to get a few answers for herself. After canceling more than one appointment with her doctor to explore the new possibilities, she faced him with her questions and her situation. He referred her to a psychiatrist, and she was faced with her next hurdle. But, having started the process, she was determined now to carry it through.

Lisa does not go without depressive episodes today. The Ominous Presence still visits her, but much less frequently than before, and her new medication does its job as well as can be expected.

Recently, Lisa began to wonder if she might be able to help other folks who suffer as she has for so long. Then she was asked to co-facilitate a group support meeting.

Am I ready for this? she asked herself. *Well, maybe I am. Maybe it's worth a try. There's only one way to find out.*

Section 3:

Reflection and Inspiration

Neither Friend Nor Foe

Trapped

One word by itself can kill,
For in the secret thoughts of a locked mind
It explodes,
And grasps to find meaning.
Unable to break the rusty locks of time,
It dies down—unshared, and not understood.

I wrote this poem when I was deeply depressed at the age of 18. I showed it to no one at the time, as I feared others would see me as I saw myself: poisonous, useless, tormented, and rotting in a black, bottomless pit. For many years, I experienced (and labeled) my depressions as "cancer of the mind," with all the horror that term arouses.

The particular words we use to describe depression and manic-depression (uni- and bi-polar disorders) can have a strong bearing on our attitude towards our potential healing or demise. Those words I used as a teenager almost brought about my own death.

I recently read an article by an American psychiatrist who referred to depression as a "dragon" and a "challenging foe" that we "try to defeat with pharmacological weapons."

I reacted strongly to his choice of terms and sent a letter to the editor of the magazine in which the article appeared.

This is what I wrote.

As a person with a 35-year history of uni-polar mood disorder, I would like to offer a different perspective on our use of language for this illness.

At one time, I too thought of depression as a savage beast that I must try to obliterate, as a red-hot dragon that I must flee from, as a deadly demon that I must annihilate with drugs. And, indeed, I have tried every weapon at one time or another: intelligent reasoning, spirituality, will power, and medication. I have even tried to bribe it.

Sadly, none of these techniques had any long-lasting, positive effect on the sorry state of any particular episode. These attempts did not help me conquer depression, nor make the enemy retreat. In fact, at times these activities directed against a foe seemed to fuel the fire of depression. I would end up feeling like a failure—a loser in this impossible fight. My feeling of self-worth would be diminished, if not demolished.

In recent times, I have tried to view my episodes differently. Rather than using provocative words (such as dragon and foe), I now use words that, to me, acutely describe the intensity of the experience, admitting to its awful reality, without giving depression the power of an enemy. I now use terms such as "the Dark Pit," and "the Ominous Presence." Admittedly, these are not exactly emotionally stripped terms. However, with the Dark Pit, I have limited success in wrapping depression into a shape that has dimensions less than infinity. With the Ominous Presence, I acknowledge its omni-present darkness, without bestowing it with hate.

In recent times when I have become depressed, I try to remind myself that I have a bio-chemical brain anomaly, some faulty wiring that causes intolerable pain. (Given the nature of the disorder, however, I cannot believe these facts while I'm in an episode.) I try to hold on to the fact that being depressed is not my fault (though it is my brain's flaw). I try to remember that the real gap in my life during an episode is that of the synapses in my brain.

I've been learning to view the seeming monster as something I must (unfortunately) live with, respond to, and, I believe, respect (I no longer pretend it isn't with me). I must "own" my body chemistry. I can't go back to the proverbial blackboard and re-design myself and start again. Depression is in me and of me. I am trying to love myself in spite of this hardship and the despair it brings. It seems to me that it is contradictory to both love myself and to seek to defeat an enemy within at the same time.

Until medications are able to deal with every twist and turn of depression, I feel I must accept the presence of this unwelcome, permanent resident in my body. I will try to shed at least a modicum of healing light on the irrepressible blackness. I will attempt to counter-balance depression's brute strength with my "weapons" of self-acceptance, patience, and trust in my close friends and family.

This is what works best for me after years of searching for language to help me live with this illness.

Making Up is Hard to Do

It had been "just another" episode, and now it was over. At least Lindsay was quite sure that it was over. Past experience had taught her, "It's not over 'til it's over." People thought she was being pessimistic when she said that. "I'm realistic," she would reply dryly, as she had been overly optimistic more than once when coming out of an episode.

Take her depression three years ago. At one point in her recovery, she thought she could go back to work and take an evening course and rejoin her tennis league. So she scheduled all three, and collapsed after just two weeks. She didn't yet have the inner resources to tackle all three at once.

So, with great reluctance, she gave up her evening course, which disappointed her immensely, begged out of her tennis commitment, for which she felt a flop, and concentrated on being back at work. Even that meant she had to rest every evening for the next month.

Gradually—only gradually—was she able to blend in other activities. It took her a full four months to be truly functional again.

What particularly annoyed and disappointed Lindsay about this failure was that she had desperately wanted to catch up on all her activities the minute she began to feel better, to make up for all that "wasted time" when she was ill.

Ah, well. That was then.

Today, Lindsay was feeling much more positive about her recovery and upcoming life. Her energy had improved daily for a good month, and her intellect was finally intact. She had successfully made her way out of the dark pit once more. *Just to be safe, I'll start out this time by only working on the stained glass window I couldn't finish because of that dumb episode. When that's done, I'll look for work.*

She was pleased with her wise plan.

She enthusiastically dove into her waiting stained glass window project, but after working for only an hour, she needed to nap.

This shouldn't be, she lamented. *I'm only doing one thing, not three, this time. I should be able to work at this for three hours at a go. That's the least I would do before my episode.*

She was beginning to feel a bit discouraged.

Over the next few days, no matter how hard she tried, she could not work for more than an hour at a time. She wondered if other people had this problem, and, decided to return to her support group to find out.

The following week, Lindsay went to the meeting. When it was her time to say how the past week had been for her, she explained her situation, looking for a simple solution.

"And this shortage of energy surprises you?" someone asked.

"Of course it does. I'm supposed to be better now."

"What does being better mean to you?" the group facilitator asked.

That's a pretty silly question, Lindsay thought, but answered politely, "It means being able to do as much now as I did before my episode. It means making up for all that lost time when I couldn't do anything."

Several people nodded in agreement. Her definition was obviously common to many people with mood disorders.

After a short while, a quiet voice said, "Shall I tell you something that I discovered?" The voice belonged to Chris.

"Yes, please!" Lindsay turned in Chris's direction.

"Well, I discovered that in fact I hadn't really, totally lost those many months when I was in my episode."

This sounded very unlikely to Lindsay.

Chris went on. "No question that when I'm in terrible mental pain, and have no energy or grey matter to do anything with, I feel I'm losing valuable life time. But, during an episode about five years ago, I did have a few calm times when I felt a bit less than dreadful and had an ounce of energy. On a few days I would walk to a quiet coffee shop, half listen to the peaceful music, and munch on a muffin. That may not seem like doing much, but I really found that it rejuvenated me, sort of nurtured my inner space."

Oh, no, thought Lindsay. *I'm not into this inner business. I'm a doer.*

"After a while I realized I was being kind to myself. That's a real accomplishment when I'm depressed. I'm not usually good to myself."

Being kind to yourself and depressed. Sounds like an oxymoron to me, Lindsay thought.

Chris ignored Lindsay's raised eyebrows and continued.

"So, I tried to do that almost every day when I was ill. And, surprise of surprises, I found that I came to a new, calmer home place when I fully recovered. I've been trying to visit that quiet, calm place almost every day since, and it's been very good for me." Chris paused, then added, "So, when I was sick and thought I wasn't doing anything, in fact something very positive was going on in me, and still continues."

Lindsay was a bit skeptical, but didn't say anything.

Chris added, almost philosophically, "Sometimes the best action is non-action."

No one in the group said anything for a few moments. There was something to think about in what Chris had just said. Lindsay looked at the floor, wondering whether she could get into non-action.

Then Trevor spoke up. "I found out something quite different than Chris did when I looked at that making-up-time problem."

"What was that?" Lindsay didn't know whether to be hopeful or not.

"I discovered that I simply can't make up for all that so-called lost time."

Lindsay groaned. *I don't want to listen to this. I ask for a simple "how," and he tells me "no way."*

Trevor interrupted Lindsay's thoughts. "When I finally accepted this fact, I was free to recover truly, gradually. And, it turns out, my recoveries since then have been quicker than those following my earlier episodes. Part of this is accepting that this illness is a reality in my ongoing life."

Lindsay was not completely convinced.

"Sounds to me like you've just given in to it," someone said sarcastically.

137

"Not at all. I feel stronger now than when I was fighting it. I just do my best with it, not against it. My life is mostly satisfying in spite of my recurring depressions."

Silence fell on the group. Everyone in the circle obviously found something to digest from what Chris and Trevor had just said. They were clearly affected by these rather unusual, and unlikely, responses to a seemingly straightforward query.

As for Lindsay, she wondered whether the issue she had brought with her this evening had been twisted around.

No, she decided. *It was just addressed in ways I would never have guessed. Certainly gives me a few new things to think about.*

Preparing for Next Time

I've always avoided anticipating my next depressive episode for fear that even contemplating it might cause it to come on sooner. Hence, I have entered each next time somewhat ill prepared, and I struggle with it, and myself, as in past times.

I am going to try to change that because during my most recent episode I almost shamed myself when I was in the spiral going down, and I wasted a lot of time during the long climb up.

In my work life I am a contract business and technical writer. By working on contract, rather than full-time, I am able to work while I am well, and bow out when I am in, or better yet, just entering an episode. At least that's how the theory goes.

Two years ago, when I was in the midst of a five-month contract, I started to feel intellectually fuzzy. I became forgetful, and somewhat scattered; my confidence sank. I truly wondered if I was up to this project. But I carried on stubbornly.

"I've done this work before. I just need to try harder," I tried to convince myself.

As luck would have it, the client cancelled the project, just as I was reaching the point where I could not have put one more paragraph together sensibly. Just in time. No harm done. But too close for comfort.

Following my lengthy down time, it took me another long time to be able to work competently. I doubted my capabilities and worried about not being able to catch up with technical advances in my field. I was mentally paralyzed for a couple of months.

When, with great nervousness, I risked re-entering the working world. I found, to my delight, once again, that I did indeed have what it takes to do my work.

Now I am safely back on track again with work and other activities, enjoying renewed confidence and self-esteem, and a new, challenging work project.

Now I have to ask myself how I could do things differently with respect to my work as I descend into and climb out of a next episode.

The descent

For me, entering an episode may be slow and almost imperceptible, or quick and painfully obvious, or somewhere in between. It's easy to conclude that a job is beyond my capabilities when in fact it is the disorder that is making the work impossible. So, how about a "barometer" to measure my intellectual capability now and then?

I could devise a test that I could administer to myself periodically that would indicate whether I was "firing on all cylinders." I could assign myself a hypothetical technical writing task. If it proved too difficult, I could take a closer look at why that was so.

A poor result would not necessarily mean that I was entering an episode. Excessive stress or family concerns are well-accepted reasons for not thinking clearly. If I weren't going through those types of worries though, there would be grounds for looking further.

I could take one of the well-known depression inventory tests, such as the often-prescribed Beck Depression Inventory, which would either support or dispute my earlier test results. If I measured high on that inventory, I could address my work life before it became a crisis.

The problem is not that I don't trust my own judgment. I don't heed it, and the formal structure of the barometers might prove more compelling. It is critical that I catch myself before my mental disabilities have destroyed my work reputation.

The climb

Coming out of an episode is essentially a happy event. Clarity returns to my mind. The world, with all its adventures and invitations, opens up again in front of me.

But remnants of the episode still have their grip. Self-doubt still intrudes. I don't know what I am capable of doing. My last period of good health seems so far back. What I remember most clearly in my awakening mind is the recent, real impossibility of working properly. I contemplate new work.

"I couldn't do that six months ago," I argue with myself. "How can I expect to do it now?"

Rather than living for months with self-doubt and the low self-esteem that accompanies it, I could again administer a depression inventory test. And on my own, I could try a work task, one untinged by the grief of my disintegrating mind during the downslide. The results of these tests would fairly accurately tell me whether I was ready for the rigors of work life again.

It's untested

Such is my new theory. I've not tried these strategies, as, fortunately, my "next time" has not yet arrived. Until it does, I am faced with many questions.

How likely is it that I will really face a downslide before I have done everything in my power to prove it's not happening? Will my pride get in the way? Will I think I'm a weakling, just giving in to an episode? Might I try to get out of a job I don't want to do by ensuring a high score on the depression inventory? Might I resist feeling better knowing that I have to face my co-workers and work full days again?

My answer to these questions right now is simply, "I don't know."

What do you think? Do you have some workable techniques that you can employ right now? Or do you do as I have done in the past; wait until it's almost too late?

Take a Hike

It wasn't Jane's idea, but she went along with it anyway, and there she was, with two pals, half way up a small mountain a few miles from town.

Jane was just coming out of a nasty depressive episode.

Am I going to swing into a manic phase in the next few weeks? she wondered.

The possibility frightened her, but she trusted that her new medication would help prevent that. Besides, she couldn't afford to speculate about going manic. She needed all her mental energy to bring herself those last few feet out of the Perilous Pit.

The horrid magnet was still trying to pull her downwards, but she knew she could now actively help herself back to wellness again. Although her brain chemistry determined when a particular episode was over, she knew that by exerting effort and taking risks again (two of her recuperating strategies), she could make her comeback shorter and less painful.

This coming-out-of-the-depths phase of her cycle was always bumpy, but at least during this time Jane got glimpses of new possibilities, of returning to school and to her hobbies. Recovery often meant new insights and clarity, but it was always countered with too many moments of returning darkness, though these did become shorter as she got better.

The experience of many episodes had not made the return to health any easier each time, but Jane knew if she was diligent and was kind to herself, good mental health could again be hers.

This was one of those days requiring much diligence. The Ominous Presence, the formidable foe with which she contends in the depths of depression and in the process of recovery, was trying to exert its dark influence on her mind.

As the hikers came to the second plateau on their trek, Jane thought, *I'm such a lousy hiker. Chris and Lee are so much more fit than I am. They choose the best activities for fitness: hiking, kayaking, and skiing, where you exercise lots of muscles, and you get great scenery to boot. All I do is swim and run the city streets. There's nothing to look at when I swim except a straight line at the bottom of the pool, and I have to fight for a lane. As far as running goes...* She caught herself mid-sentence.

Let go of that, she reminded herself. *Thinking like that will only make trouble.*

She had learned this let-go-of-that routine from a woman in her support group, and she had had modest success with it. All you had to do (<u>All</u> you had to do?) was to gently stop negative thoughts about yourself as soon as you recognized them.

So Jane cleared her mind of those self-deprecating thoughts and brought her mind back to the hike. She took a deep breath and looked around at the fresh-leafed maples.

May in the forest is like me these days. Coming out of an episode is like spring time with its warming weather, and newness, and its surprising snow storms. I'm definitely in one of those stupid storms today.

"Look at this saprophyte," Chris exclaimed. "I haven't seen one of these in years!"

What the hell is a saprophyte? How come I missed that? Pay attention. Get with it.

Oops, she had fallen in the trap again. More negative thoughts about herself.

Let go of that, she reminded herself.

Further along the path, Lee asked Jane, "What did you think of that natural bridge back there?"

She hadn't even seen the bridge though they had all walked across it. She had been busy chastising herself for not knowing the names of any of the wildflowers they had passed.

I don't know anything, she had been thinking when Lee interrupted her thoughts.

Let go of that, she reminded herself.

"Oh," she replied to Lee's question, "it was neat." She was hoping that that was a suitable response.

Jane was getting discouraged by her mind, which seemed to gravitate towards negative statements about herself.

There must be a better way to deal with this. I'm not faring very well today. The Ominous Presence is scoring a lot better than I am.

144

A better way. A better way, she repeated to herself, trying to coax her mind into a better way of dealing with this negativity, this pre-occupation, when she should be completely in the outdoors, on this hike, with her pals.

All of a sudden, out of the blue, Jane remembered the meditation course she took last year. She had stopped meditating once the course was over, but she did remember the teacher saying more than once, "It's a matter of being here now."

Yes, that was the basic message. Be aware of what is going on at this moment. Use a word to help keep that awareness if that is helpful. And when your mind wanders, just bring it back to what is going on at the moment.

It had sounded, at the time, like good advice, and something that should be fairly easy to do, but she'd found it harder than she'd thought. She could "be here now" for only about two consecutive seconds by the end of the course, so she'd stopped practicing.

But I could try it right this minute; it can't be any worse than what I have been doing.

Walking, walking, Jane slowly and silently repeated to herself to help her remain aware of what she was doing.

Hey, that's a neat sound, she thought as she listened to the sounds of her boots on the cushy earth. *But why should I have to do this silly meditating stuff? Chris and Lee don't have to. I'm so retarded.*

Walking, walking. Jane gently brought her mind back to what she was doing. She was getting excited about the changing scenery. *Hey, look at the distinct shapes of the different plants. I've never noticed that so much before. I wish I could keep this awareness forever. But, if you've got this stupid illness, you can't expect that. It's so hard to just let life be. I bet Chris doesn't have to do this.*

Walking, Walking. Jane gently brought her mind back to what she was doing and noticed that her breathing was becoming heavier as they climbed.

Hey, I like that rhythm of my breathing. I feel like I am in sync with the forest. But Lee doesn't seem to be breathing heavily. I must be in worse shape than I thought.

Walking, walking. Jane gently brought her mind back to what she was doing...

By the end of the day's hike, she had gently brought her mind back to what she was doing at least three hundred times, she guessed. She decided to do an assessment.

Did I have a more enjoyable hike because I did that meditating bit?

Of course she couldn't know the answer for sure, but when she cast her mind back over the hike, she found she was left with a feeling that was much more positive than negative.

I guess those monks knew what they were doing after all. Maybe I'll try it again sometime.

Waiting and Waiting

Those of us who experience episodes of depression usually find them painful, frustrating, frightening, and isolating. As if that's not bad enough, while we are in the throes of an episode and desperately want to get out of the darkness, we are forced to wait. We have to wait for medication to take effect. We have to wait for our mood to lift. We have to wait for our energy to return. We have to wait for our intellect to get back to normal. That's a lot of waiting.

What do we mean by "wait?" How best can we wait? What can we do while we wait?

Wait means different things to different people in different circumstances. The basic implication in "waiting" is the passage of time. If we don't have to wait to have something, we can have it now. If we don't have to wait to do something, we can do it now. Time, at least, is not holding us back.

People have different approaches and attitudes to waiting, and they do different things when they have to wait. Consider standing on a street corner, waiting for a bus. People in this situation might:

- Walk briskly to the next stop, hoping to arrive there before the bus does.
- Stand at the bus stop and stare down the street to where the bus will eventually become visible, as if their fixed gaze will hasten its arrival.
- Twirl their umbrellas or shuffle their feet, indicating that their frustration threshold is fast approaching.
- Become angry at the bus, the bus driver, and, if they have to wait a very long time, the entire bus company. When the bus finally arrives, their anger may be turned towards the person in front of them in the line up who took the last seat.
- Read a newspaper or magazine; daydream; think about what they might get a friend for her birthday; chat to the stranger next to them.

Clearly some of the ways in which people wait for a bus are constructive, some are destructive, and some are just a matter of putting in (some would say wasting) time. The reality is that if you

147

want to catch a particular bus, you may have to wait, and waiting for even five minutes can present a challenge to your patience.

For those of us who experience recurring depression, there are times when we <u>must</u> wait, times when we <u>should</u> wait, and times when we <u>must not</u> or <u>should not</u> wait but do so anyway. We need to know when it is appropriate to wait, and when it is mandatory to act.

We should not wait in dread of our next episode when we are in perfectly good health. We must live fully and meaningfully while we are well.

When symptoms of depression appear, we should not wait to address them. They have a tendency to gather momentum, like a toboggan gaining speed as it goes downhill. We can't always avert an episode even if we act quickly, but the possibility, however remote, is there if we do act and not if we don't.

If an episode is inevitable, we should not just wait to hit rock bottom. We should do those things that simplify our lives, give us comfort, help us to feel safe. We may employ strategies that helped during our previous episode: tell family and close friends about our difficulties, make lists of things we must do each day, make sure we have recorded for ourselves our passwords for the bank, for our computers, and so on. We must remember, too, that while we are administering this necessary self-help, we need to remain open to the possibility that this episode could recede at any time.

When we are in the depths of an episode, we must continue to take good care of ourselves, do whatever we can to feel secure, look after our vulnerabilities, and generally make life as tolerable as possible. In the midst of our darkness, despair, and self-care, we wait. We wait for the darkness to lift; we wait for our vulnerabilities to fade and our fears to disappear; we wait for any sign that tells us good mental health is again a possibility for us.

While we are waiting and waiting, someone may say to us, "This too will pass," or some other maxim that is meant to be inspirational. Unfortunately, these words may have the opposite effect and upset us, depressing us further when we cannot imagine an end to our agony. But the person who offers us the maxim is often sincere and caring, and the maxim is true. The episode will pass some day, some week, or some month hence. Our supporters want to encourage us during our waiting, and they wait, as we do, for our good health to return.

There are many different approaches and attitudes to waiting for an episode to end, some negative and some positive.

The negative approaches may be something like the following:

- We can try to run away from our depression, by rushing and pushing ourselves towards good health, pretending we aren't in the episode. This often exacts a heavy price, as episodes have their own timetables, and those timetables are never revealed to us.

- We can chase from one activity to another. But in doing this we risk becoming confused, exhausted, and discouraged. In our vulnerable state, we may encounter any number of situations that make us feel worse than we already do.

- We may "twiddle our thumbs." This is often difficult to do for any length of time during an episode. Just sitting for a long time when we're depressed doesn't necessarily stop our mind from tormenting us. Staring out the window or at a wall may be comforting for a while, but eventually we return to our own heads and our depression.

- After months, or even only weeks, of depression, we may become very frustrated and angry at the waste of valuable living time. We turn our anger towards ourselves, our families and friends, and even (or especially) at the medical system that hasn't yet figured out how to cure our illness. Such anger is understandable, but not productive.

I'm sure you know of, and may even have experienced, other ways of waiting unproductively.

The positive or productive approaches are more difficult, but they do exist. As hard as it may be to imagine, let alone accomplish, we can try to wait with some faith that good health will return. We can attempt to be patient.

But how do we do this? What do we do while we are waiting, when we feel despondent, useless to our families, friends, and the world in general?

- We can take good care of ourselves. We can do what we have to do to feel safe. If we feel frightened of being alone, we may choose to go to a library, or walk in a busy park, where we may feel safer with other people around.

• We can be kind and polite to other people, especially those who support us emotionally. We need as much love, care, and comfort as we can get when we are ill, but it is all too easy to strike out in pain at those close to us. This hurts everyone.

• We can maintain reasonably good physical health by eating properly, by getting enough sleep (taking one or more naps during the day if necessary), and by exercising (even if it means just walking around inside our home once a day).

• We can formulate and employ useful strategies for getting through each day. Make a list of when to take how much of which medication. Establish a routine that works well. We may choose to reread an inspirational work that has helped us during earlier episodes. We may even have written down special passages and have them handy to read when we are feeling particularly despondent.

• We should do those things that give even momentary relief from our pain, as long as they don't cause harm to ourselves or to others. Go to a movie in the afternoon. Have salad for breakfast and porridge for dinner, if that is comforting to us.

• It helps if we can find even one small something that makes us feel useful each day. It could be emptying the dishwasher, or taking the recycling out, or some other task that requires minimal thought and energy.

It is almost impossible for me to do anything smoothly or properly when I'm deeply depressed. Sometimes all I can do is make batches of scrap paper out of used computer paper. I cut a stack of the used paper in two, making all the sheets 5.5 inches by 8.5 inches. I then staple about ten sheets together, blank side up. Voila! My task is complete, and I feel a tiny bit better, if only for a minute. It's not much of an achievement under normal conditions, but it helps to know that I can do *something* useful when I'm depressed.

Besides, it provides me with lots of paper on which I can write reminders that are essential when I am in an episode.

Having to wait five months for an episode to lift makes having to wait five minutes for a bus seem trivial. But we can make waiting for the end of an episode more bearable by finding ways to help ourselves during that time. We can make the long wait worth something.

From Nervous to Enthused

I visited my hairdresser today. Natalie and I always chat while she's cutting my hair, and today our conversation turned to smoking. It's an easy topic for me. I was addicted to smoking in my twenties and was able to quit for good about 15 years ago.

Natalie talked about her 21-year-old daughter who smokes a pack a day. Never having smoked herself, Natalie cannot understand why Rebecca won't quit.

Rebecca says, "I want to, Mom, but I can't. I just can't go to those quit-smoking clinics. I get all sweaty just thinking of it."

That was exactly how I felt for the year before I quit, and I found myself being drawn towards actively supporting Rebecca in her bid to stop smoking.

I had met this young woman once and found her to be very personable. But it wasn't as if she were my sister or daughter or close friend. I was taken aback by my eagerness to help.

When I decided to give up smoking, I tried various courses, gimmicks, and products. What turned out to be most instrumental to my success was the BC Lung Association program. I mentioned it to Natalie, suggesting she pass it on to Rebecca. I added that if Rebecca had questions but felt shy about calling the association, I would be happy to talk with her about it.

After I left Natalie's place, I wondered why Rebecca is so reticent about going to a quit-smoking group. I looked back to earlier times in my own life.

When I decided long ago to join the BC Lung group, I was nervous. I didn't know what to expect. What do other aspiring-to-quit smokers look like? Do they have their mouths taped so they can't smoke? Do they have cigarettes growing out their ears so they can smoke? Do they have no fingernails left?

Yes, I was nervous. It hadn't occurred to me that other going-to-be non-smokers might be nervous like me, look like me, wear lipstick like I do, and use their ears for hearing.

Similarly, when I went to my first Adult Children of Alcoholics meeting, I felt apprehensive. I didn't know what to expect. Would everyone look all beat up? Would they be untrusting? Would they be intolerant of anyone who sometimes takes a drink?

Yes, I went with some uncertainty. It hadn't occurred to me that adult children of alcoholics might look like me (weary but not beat up), want to trust people who seem reliable, and have a glass of sherry now and then.

And finally, when I went to my first Mood Disorders Association meeting six years ago as a person with a hereditary bio-chemical brain irregularity, I was downright terrified. I didn't know what to expect. What do people with mood disorders look like? Do they cry all the time? Are they constantly looking for a tall building to leap from? Will they crumble if I say "hello?"

Yes, I was very scared. It hadn't occurred to me that other people who have mood disorders might look like me, wear jeans one day and a suit the next as I do, enjoy the revolving restaurants in some tall buildings as I do. And guess who was the one who felt like crumbling?

There are dozens of special interest support groups in every province and state, including 12-step programs, single moms groups, families of victims of violence, parents of children in trouble, to name a few, and I had gone to three of them.

I'd gone with considerable anxiety, and in fact I almost didn't get to any of them on account of wracked nerves. But all of them worked out very well for me, very much to my advantage in the long term.

I was so fearful back then, before each of my excursions, as I suspect most other first-timers are. But, after having attended these groups for a while, I found I had to calm my enthusiasm so I wouldn't frighten potential participants away. Why couldn't I have been less nervous then and less ardent now?

In order to even consider going to any of these programs, I had to muster the courage to accept parts of myself that had been hurt or that I had denied. I had to be humble enough to seek help. I was afraid of the unknowns. Would I be taking a major step towards becoming who I really wanted to be, or naturally am, or would I fall flat on my face? These are no small questions.

Having embarked on these various journeys, I found other people welcoming and helpful, and I discovered how successful group support can be. I found out I wasn't alone in my pursuit of authenticity, and that breaking new ground is not only necessary, but also sometimes fun. And fun usually leads to enthusiasm.

I have turned from being a frightened outsider to one who believes firmly in these three organizations and who continues to participate in two of them. What I do now is watch out for nervous or frightened souls who stand at the door, wondering how they could possibly come in, and quietly extend my hand.

Two out of Three

About a year ago, Patrick entered one of those all too familiar episodes. It was springtime. New life and levity and happy days on the golf course with his pals are meant to happen during the greening season.

But Patrick's brain chemistry has a mind of its own, a fact he had only recently, reluctantly, come to accept. He knows now that he cannot choose whether or when to have these episodes.

Accustomed to his own particular pattern of depressive cycles, Patrick knows that one of three things announces the onset of a downer.

- The physical, mental, emotional, and spiritual energy begins to drain out of him, slowly but surely. It drains from so many places. Attempts to plug the innumerable escape hatches are fruitless. He feels as heavy as a concrete block, as agile as a rhinoceros.

- His mood darkens gradually, with no apparent reason. Imperceptible at first, it soon becomes a minor, then major, problem. As he descends into the deep black pit, his self-confidence and self-esteem almost disintegrate, and he feels alone in this closing-in world.

- His mind becomes hazy. He finds concentrating increasingly difficult. Work is no longer a challenge. It is an impossibility. The haze worsens until he has trouble adding 2 and 2, which for an engineer is a serious problem.

Whatever the first sign is, his attempts to turn things around are fruitless, and the slide continues.

When Patrick is entering an episode, but not sure that his problems are internal, he questions every aspect of his external life.

What am I doing wrong that makes me feel so bad? Is my relationship not going well? Am I under excessive stress at work? Is this a mid-life crisis?

He searches for an external precipitator in vain, reluctant to acknowledge the mood disorder he has housed all his life.

Eventually, he experiences all three symptoms. He bottoms out and finds himself in hell once more. He knows he has no strength to fight the Ominous Presence, that most horrible of uninvited guests. So, he gives in and subsists in emotional, mental, and spiritual pain for months.

* * *

During this most recent episode, however, things didn't go as usual. The first symptom struck. This time it was mental confusion. Patrick was unable to work with his usual acuity and that worried him a great deal. Once again, he wondered whether he just didn't have what it takes to be an engineer after all.

Was I expecting too much of myself by taking on this career? Is this particular project too tough for me?

The second symptom, the energy drain, came along about a month later.

Maybe I don't like spring after all; maybe I have a thyroid condition; maybe I should get more sleep.

Finally, after exhausting all other possibilities, Patrick realized where he was going: down the razor slide to the most dreaded possible place.

He knew that the plummeting mood would come along soon. He waited and waited.

There wasn't much he could do but wait, take his medication, inform friends and family about his changing state, and try to implant somewhere in his disordered mind, that "this too will pass."

He became more intellectually confused and had to take time off work. He was spending more time lying exhausted on his bed each day. He dragged himself about the house as if he weighed 400 pounds. And he couldn't remember, 15 minutes after having done so, whether he had let the dog out.

But after a month of combined fatigue and mental morass, Patrick's mood still didn't plummet. He continued to wait but it didn't happen.

It will, he assured himself.

But after another two months, it hadn't. This was incredible. He had always experienced, at some point during an episode, the unmanageable triad of energy loss, mental confusion, and darkest of moods.

He was amazed and tremendously thankful, but also dubious.

Why haven't I yet been tormented by the Ominous Presence? Is it lurking around the corner, just waiting for its perfect time to strike?

Six months passed. Patrick's energy began to recover. He returned to work. His self-confidence and self-esteem improved slowly, with much nurturing. It was a very rough period, but not as bad as usual.

It wasn't until he was back working competently, playing squash, and spending time with friends again, that he could trust that the Ominous Presence wouldn't knock him over this time.

Why was it different for this episode? Could it be the new medication? Did my brain decide to take it easy on me this time?

Patrick doesn't know. He doesn't think anyone really knows. Whatever the case, he feels fortunate. His unexpected experience gave new meaning to one of his favourite old hit songs: "Two out of three ain't bad."

Yes, I Will

I used to interpret the saying, "Where there's a will, there's a way" very narrowly. I believed that if I willed something—anything—if I really wanted it, and if I exerted sufficient effort and perseverance pursuing it, I could achieve it.

But when I tried to put this belief into practice during an episode of depression, I was, more often than not, discouraged, disappointed, and angry with myself at my lack of success.

There are times for many or most of us when we devoutly aspire to ideals that are impossible to achieve. For instance, if I willed myself to be rid of my depressive illness, I would have as little chance at success as a diabetic willing himself to be rid of diabetes.

Though neither illness can be willed away, or, to date, be cured, both can be successfully treated—depressive illness with anti-depressants or mood stabilizers or both, and with psychotherapy; diabetes with insulin, other medication, or with weight loss and diet control.

We who experience depression over and over again sometimes feel cheated and frustrated.

If we will ourselves not to have another episode, we fail. Then we may will the episode to be brief, only to be disheartened and angered by its lingering presence. By willing something that is impossible, we risk losing confidence in ourselves, our medical advisors, and the world in general.

In order to deal effectively with our illness, we must look very carefully and candidly at it when we are well. We must understand and accept where our illness takes us and what it's like to be there, before we can begin to make appropriate adjustments and improvements.

My analysis of my situation is all I can offer. While I know that it will differ in some respects from yours, I'm confident that my thinking will be similar to yours at many points.

Despite my best intentions and my excellent medical care, I continue to have episodes of depression. My psychiatrists and I have yet to find a combination of medications that will banish any chance of future episodes. There has always been, to date anyway, a next time.

In the past, when, despite my will against it, I have bumped into that next time, I have thought, "It's all my fault. If I had done this, or not done that, I wouldn't be facing an episode." This perception only pushed me more quickly towards the painful place that I call "The Dark Pit." My self-contempt for letting the episode in, if not bringing it on, became carved in stone.

These thoughts and feelings are very difficult to dispel, but although they still reign in my bad times, I can now suspend or even surmount them during my good times, and I have concluded that it is both unrealistic and unwise for me to will myself to never have another episode.

I know now that I must redirect my will towards seeking the best available treatment and maintaining it to the best of my ability, and towards fuller appreciation of the good times and more prudent and sympathetic preparation for the bad times.

To this end, I can will myself early on in an episode to have the courage, patience, and inner strength to endure this very tough time. My will-power may not obliterate or shorten the episode, but it might positively affect the way I experience the dark and desolate time.

During my most recent episode, I couldn't successfully will myself to not feel isolated and afraid in the afternoon, my time of deepest agony when I'm depressed. I was able though, to will myself to approach the afternoons with more care and wisdom.

I could ensure that I was not alone, even if it meant going to the library or sitting in a coffee shop for two hours. Although my afternoons were by no means enjoyable, I had made them less isolating and frightening. I had found a way to feel safer at a time when I usually feel most vulnerable and cut off from the world.

Physical exhaustion is another characteristic common to most of my depressive episodes. I no longer will myself to have as much energy when I'm ill as I have when I'm well. Rather, I vow to do the best I can with what I have.

When I'm well, I can run six miles with little difficulty, but I can barely walk 25 yards when I'm ill. It is not realistic to pledge to run even half a mile when I'm depressed, but I can promise myself that I will exercise as much as I can, even if it's just a five-minute walk each day.

Setting goals is closely related to will-power, even dependent upon it. Those of us with episodes of depression need, as other people do, a set of goals to strive for when we are in good mental health. We base these on our "normal" intellectual and physical capabilities, and we select new goals based on the success we have had in reaching our earlier ones.

When we are depressed, these goals often become impractical.

I have always wanted to learn to golf and have set a date by which I hope to be a proficient player. I will need to alter this goal if my learning is interrupted by a depressive episode. This reality is disappointing, but if I don't adjust to accommodate my state of health, I will become frustrated, probably more depressed, and may utterly fail to learn the game. In fact, I could well come to hate it.

If, when I'm depressed, I adjust my goals accordingly, I am more likely to continue to pursue and reach them when I am well again, and less likely to feel guilty for not reaching them when I am ill.

I also set specific, practical, and, I hope, realistic goals for myself when I sense that I am entering an episode. I can, for example, give myself the challenge of doing one useful thing each day. It might be something as simple as taking out the garbage, or setting the table, but it must be something that I know is physically and mentally reachable during an episode.

If I succeed, my depression doesn't lift, but I do feel better, if only for a moment or two, because of my effort, my self-discipline, my self-will.

Three Times and She's Almost Out

She thought that by now she would be used to it. After all, she had already "come out" twice in her thirty years. This time didn't feel much easier, and she wondered why.

These were her "invisible impediments" as she had labeled them.

She had known since she was eleven that she was not exactly her father's child. Mom had told her tearfully (and, it turned out, regrettably) shortly after Dad had died. It had to do with someone coming to town when Dad was working overseas.

She was...oh my God, could she mouth it? Well... she was illegitimate. She hated that awful word.

She had loved the Dad she had known very much, but the terrible fact of her beginnings tormented her throughout her teens. She had felt horribly ashamed and guilty, so had shared this dark and sordid truth with absolutely no one.

She'd realized in her twenties that guarding this unsavory secret was driving her crazy. She'd concluded that she would have to release it in order to regain some sense of sanity.

The main obstacle to disclosing the truth was her intense fear of rejection. But when she'd finally told some friends of her reality (she couldn't mouth the "i" word, much less the "b" word), no one had rejected her. In fact they had all been warm and understanding.

She'd felt better after revealing her secret, but she hadn't felt complete relief.

A few years later, when she was comfortable with others knowing who she was (or, more accurately, who she wasn't), she had recognized that it was time to deal with her second secret. Only her Mom knew about this one: her long, dark, deep bouts of depression.

She would put on a happy face for her friends when she was feeling confused, in dread, and isolated. Then she would go home and cry inconsolably on her bed for hours. After having recovered from several of these horrible descents, she'd realized once again that in order to live with herself, she would have to be honest with her closest friends. She would have to reveal her dark secret.

I've been here once before, she had thought confidently. *This should be easier than the first time.*

Her friends had been compassionate. They had asked what they could do to help her when she was down. *It was easier than the first time.*

But having disclosed the second secret, she hadn't felt "clean," "visible," or even "okay."

Why not? I've been honest and open, haven't I? Oh well... I've dealt with two debilitating secrets now. Time to get on with life.

In time though, she had realized that she was confined to a third closet, one she hadn't recognized as a closet before.

She had always considered spirituality a private, secretive affair practiced only behind the closed, and preferably locked, door of one's study. Church had never been the place for her. She had assumed that one just naturally put one's spiritual books in the closet, quite literally. And she certainly couldn't have her friends associating her, even incorrectly, with groupies and fundamentalists, or with the reborn.

So, that's the secret that's been strangling me. Okay. I've done it twice before. I'll just tell the world and get it over with.

So, she had told the world, and the world had said, "That's great. We're glad you've found your path."

But again, she hadn't felt completely freed from her lonely hiding place.

She had had enough of this nonsense, of feeling guilty, ashamed, chopped up, and locked up, of still feeling ruled by her three invisible realities.

What's going on here?

As she pondered this very private, interior question, she was struck by the awareness that it was she, and not anyone else in her life, who was "bastaphobic," "moodophobic," and "spiritophobic." It was she alone who was rejecting and judgmental. In this big, strange world in which she lived, no one else was putting her down, making her hide.

At long last, she knew that her three closets were her own negative thoughts and feelings.

I've been my own worst enemy without knowing it. Finally, I'm free! Well... no, I don't feel totally free. Why? What's in my way?

She realized she had some further inner work to do.

Now I have to learn to be patient with myself. I have to untangle all this self-condemnation. I need to forgive myself for deploring myself. Then... then I'll be free. I'll be well and truly "out."

Resurfacing: A Time to Celebrate

Recovery from a depressive episode is usually not the smooth, quick climb up that we would all like it to be. We'd like each day to be better than the one before. It often isn't. We don't want recovery to take more than a week. It usually does. We'd like to control the process. We can't.

Words We Use

There are special words to describe our illness and the process of an episode of depression. When we recover from an episode, we are in fact healing. This does not mean that we are cured of the illness. No cure has yet been found for recurring depression, though many successful treatments are available, such as medications, light boxes, and psychotherapy. When we have finished healing from an episode, the best we can say is that the illness is in remission.

From my extensive experience with episodes, I am able to identify four phases in the cycle of my depressive illness. I call them wellness, declining mental health, depression itself, and recovery.

The beginning and ending of the recovery phase are very difficult to pin down. When you are coming out of an episode of depression, can you pinpoint the day your recovery began? Probably not. It no doubt seemed like one day you were convinced you were on your way "up," then the next day you fell back to feeling dreadful. That is the nature of the illness.

The process of recovery varies from person to person, and may even vary from episode to episode for one person, but there are some characteristics and distinct stages that are common to most recovery periods. Understanding these characteristics and stages won't shorten the time of our recovery, but may help to make it a little smoother, a little gentler.

Before we can improve our understanding of the recovery process, we must acknowledge that it is happening. Many people believe that they are either well or ill, and thus don't accept that there is a transitional period. But they go through it nonetheless.

Then we must acknowledge the importance of tending to our needs during recovery. We must accept that this is as important as looking after ourselves when we are well and when the early symptoms of an episode appear.

The Recovery Process

We each have our individual patterns of recovery. We may not always be able to discern the stages, and in fact, we may not go through all the stages each time. People who cycle rapidly will likely experience a different kind of recovery than those who recover gradually, over a longer period. As well, we may not seem to go through all the stages during each episode. Recovery can be very "elastic" and unpredictable, and it can be both joyful and painful at the same time.

Let us consider five stages of recovery. I have adopted my ideas from an excellent book about going through many of life's expected changes, called *Rites of Passage: Celebrating Life's Changes*, by Kathleen Wall and Gary Ferguson. It seems to me that the changes we go through as we experience cycles of depression—and mania, if we are bi-polar—are shared, to some extent, by many people as they meet the challenges of "normal" life.

You may find the following information valuable in charting your way through recovery from a depressive episode.

Stages of Recovery

Letting go

A faint, faint light appears during a lengthy period of darkness.

In this stage, we make a conscious decision to let go of the episode and create an inner feeling of readiness to open ourselves to the re-emergence of good mental health.

If we are not willing to embrace unknown possibilities, our time in darkness may be unnecessarily lengthened. Letting go requires us to risk sliding back into our depression. There are no guarantees as to what will happen when we let go, but at some point we <u>will</u> let go of the depression.

170

Wandering
The faint light goes on and off, moves to and fro, frustrates us with its inconsistency.

After deciding to embrace a healing period, we may enter a period of limbo, a time of confusion. We ask, "Where am I? I'm not where I was; I'm not where I am going," or, "I've been absent from the 'real world' for so long. How can I return to it?"

At this point, we have no clear sense of direction, and no vision of the road that lies ahead. But we sense that there is a world out there for us to re-join.

Experiencing polarities
With the light teasing us, we get pulled this way and that.

As a result of being confused during the wandering stage, we may face opposing urges, emotions, or thoughts. It's frustrating to be pulled in several directions at once. Contradictory feelings inevitably arise: anger and gladness, despair and hope. It may be very difficult for us to be decisive. We have to learn to make choices again and regain some of life's skills after being in an episode.

Beginning anew
Eventually, the light settles in one spot. We can trust it now. We feel we are entering the true light of day once again.

With our evolving experience in the "normal world" again, we get our bearings. We may see a new beginning in the midst of change. We may discover a fresh and more satisfying way of relating to the world around us. We may become excited, and at times impatient. In some ways it feels almost like a "rebirth," and on a few days we may even feel a "high".

Taking roots at a new place
The sun shines for us as it does for everyone.

With all that we have learned and absorbed in our early stages of recovery, we now say an emphatic "Yes!" to our new place in life. We can trust our return to good health. All our mental faculties and capabilities have returned to us. We can now integrate our inner vision of a new beginning into the daily realities of our life. We experience new vitality. The world welcomes us back.

Spirals, Not Cycles

Once recovered, we may feel that we lost all positive movement and growth, that we are back where we were when the slide began, when in fact we are simply at a new place.

Our subconscious has been working positively on our behalf while we've been contending with the darkness, and the world has moved along. We may even have profited from our down time by having done something new in caring for ourselves during the episode.

T. S. Eliot expressed these sentiments well in his *Four Quartets*:

> We shall not cease from exploration
> And the end of all our exploring
> Will be to arrive where we started
> And know the place for the first time.

Remnants and Closure

Stages of recovery give us a chance to deal with remnants of the episode. What we have to deal with depends on our personality, the length of the episode, the depth of our pain, and our usual expectations of ourselves.

During our episode, we likely felt one or more of the following:

- Anger at having the episode, at its timing in our lives, and at having the illness at all
- Grief over our many losses, including lost time and involvement in the world
- Resentment that others have moved ahead with their lives while we think we haven't moved at all except maybe backwards
- Guilt that we "didn't get anything done" during the episode.

When these remnants have been dealt with, we can truly say, "I am healthy once again, and I'm ready to move on." We will have given closure to the episode, and we will have the energy and clarity to start the next chapter of our lives.

A Time to Celebrate
Recovering from a bout of depression is a victory, an ending and a new beginning, a "graduation." Our struggle to regain good mental health deserves more recognition from us than, "Oh, well, it's about time," or, "Good riddance!" Since we can't skip recovery, and since we've worked hard for it, why not celebrate?

What to Celebrate
There are many things we might celebrate on our way "back up."
- Being able to get by with only one nap a day
- Being comfortable alone for several hours
- Once again visiting a friend—and enjoying it
- Being able to concentrate on a movie or book
- Being able to make a meal by ourselves
- Walking for 30 minutes
- Laughing.

Think about it. Your triumphs may be different, but they're there and they're definitely worth celebrating.

How to Celebrate
Referring back to the list of stages of recovery, we can assign a few possible celebratory activities to each stage.

The stages of recovery	Symbols for going through this stage	Examples of celebrating
Letting go	Releasing an object into the wind	Release a balloon into the air.
	Burning an object, or casting it into the water	Burn or shred any journal writings of self-hate, despair, etc. that you wrote
	Shredding, tearing,	

	cutting, or crumbling an object Burying objects in the ground	while you were depressed.
Wandering	Putting an empty vessel such as a cup, a bowl, or a vase in a special place	Place an empty plant pot in a prominent place in your bedroom. The vessel must belong to you; it need not be expensive.
Experiencing polarities	Setting out or using at the same time: Hot and cold Hard and soft Other polarities: Bitter and sweet Sunlight and shade Earth and sky Masculine and feminine	Eat hot and cold food at the same time; for instance, hot tea and ice cream. Place a rock (hard) and pillow (soft) in your study area.
Beginning anew	Planting or sowing living things Purchasing an item that is personal and meaningful	Plant seeds or seedlings in your empty pot (from the wandering stage). Buy a new outfit, the book you've always wanted, or other meaningful "treat."
Taking roots at a new place	Having a celebration	Celebrate by having a friend over for a unique dinner.

	Doing something that, for you, is fresh and untried	Go to a park, museum, or any place you've never been to before.

Clearly, there are many opportunities for celebrating. Maybe we celebrate each stage of each recovery period, or maybe we do only one thing that celebrates the end of the episode. But celebrate we must!

You and I will have different rituals. That's fine and natural. The important thing is to choose rituals that are meaningful to you.

When you are next recovering from a depressive episode, or after your next episode is over, do something special for yourself. You deserve it!

Don't Search for the Answer

It's Scott's practice these days, after being friends with a person for a while, to confess that he has a mood disorder. It usually works out okay. The new friend will respond with something like, "Oh, I wondered about those times you seemed to go out of circulation for a while," or, "That's interesting; now, as I was saying...." or, "Gosh, I'm sorry."

At times it hasn't worked out so well.

About ten years ago, Scott had a friend, Brad, whom he met at the squash club. Scott thought they understood each other pretty well. When they were in the locker room after their games, they would discuss every topic under the sun, except any health related issues, including depression, which they did not discuss at all.

At that point Scott had not told any of his friends about his disorder because he felt ashamed and guilty about his illness. He had talked about it to only one person, his brother. After being silent for so long, and feeling periodically isolated from his friends, he decided to take the risk of telling a few of them.

So who better to tell than Brad? After all, they'd been good friends for five years now.

Scott nervously raised the subject over beers one evening, and Brad's response was "I see. Yes, I understand." Words with little emotion, but Scott felt they were meant to be supportive.

That was the last time he saw or spoke with Brad. Brad's roommate screened his calls at home, and his secretary did the same at work. He changed squash clubs. Scott's good friend had abruptly severed their friendship.

Scott was both shocked and disappointed. He searched his soul for an answer to the simple question, "What drove Brad away?" Eventually, he came up with a few possibilities.

Maybe Brad realized all of a sudden that he didn't like Scott after all.

Unlikely.

Maybe he disliked anyone who seems weak and has emotional problems.

Some folks are that way.

177

Maybe Brad was unsure of his own mental health, and relating to someone who has accepted a mood distinction (as Scott liked to call it) was too close for his comfort.

There could be something to that, but how would I know?

Because he hadn't spoken to him since that last supper five years ago, Scott didn't know which of these, or other, reasons had precipitated Brad's disappearance from his life.

In the intervening years, Scott hadn't experienced such a painful curtailment, until...

A couple of years ago, a bunch of guys moved in down the street. Scott became pals with one of them, Neil. They played tennis together and did some mountain biking. Neil had a self-protective shield securely in place, but Scott knew that everyone's self-protective to a degree.

Three months ago, Scott got around to telling Neil about his mood disorder. Neil looked somewhat askance, which bothered Scott a bit.

One day recently when they were chatting, Neil's shield slipped a bit and he mentioned that a cousin of his was a schizophrenic. Then he swiftly drew back.

After that, Neil made sure that they talked about only safe matters. Several times Scott asked if he'd like to go bike-riding, but the answer was always, "Thanks, but not today. I'm too busy. But, let's do that another time."

Scott called again, but the response was always more or less the same. "I have a bunch of important chores to do. But, try me again."

He was becoming quite hurt by these rejections, and after one too many, he was propelled back to five years ago, to Brad. He was faced again with these old unanswered questions to which he added some new ones:

Does Neil think that depression and schizophrenia are contagious?

Is he ashamed and embarrassed about having a relative, and now a friend, who has a mental illness?

Is he afraid that other people might wonder why he would be friendly with this "unstable" guy?

178

This time, instead of remaining quiet, Scott asked Neil bluntly, "Does it bother you that I have a mood disorder, or that I told you I have one?"

Neil answered vaguely, "Oh, no, of course not."

This was followed by an uncomfortable silence, and then a sigh of what Scott sensed to be resignation.

That was it. Neil would say nothing more, and Scott felt very sad that he was not able to continue his companionship with a person he had considered a good friend.

He recalled what one of his favourite writers, Rainer Maria Rilke, had written to a young poet who was impatient for the answer to a personal question.

"Be patient toward all that is unsolved in your heart and try to love the *questions themselves*... Do not now seek the answers,... *Live* the questions now... Perhaps you will then gradually, without noticing it, live along some distant day into the answer."

Scott decided to take Rilke's advice.

A Hard Pill to Swallow

Brenda closes her journal, pushes herself away from her desk, and smiles. She feels a lightness, a clarity she has never known before in her 38 years. Mind you, she made sure no one was watching her as she went through her lengthy exercise in her locked study.

She leans back, stretches her legs and reflects on the strange and unlikely process that has brought her to this feeling of peace.

* * *

Brenda has experienced depressive bouts for the past 15 years. She can't remember how many episodes she's gone through, because each one was supposed to be "the final one".

After struggling on her own with debilitating downs for 10 years, she took her mom's advice to see a psychiatrist. After a few sessions, the shrink, as she liked to call him, handed her a diagnosis of uni-polar mood disorder, and a prescription for anti-depressants. Having run out of reasonable options, Brenda had the prescription filled and was starting on her second week on the pills.

I'm sure they won't work, she told herself.

She had made all sorts of assumptions and had come to all sorts of conclusions about what she had diagnosed as a character flaw. Her shrink had tried many times to set her straight on the medical definition of her problem, but Brenda had resisted any notion of disorder.

"Disorder sounds like I've got a screw missing or something," she had argued. "I know I have a character flaw because otherwise I'd be able to do something about it."

Frustrated by Brenda's intransigence, her shrink finally told her to list her assumptions about whatever it was she thought she had.

"Bring it along next time," he ordered.

That was an easy assignment. Whenever Brenda took on an assignment, in school, in extra-curricular activities, in anything, she did it with a vengeance. She had been on the debating team at college, where you had to defend a point of view even if you didn't believe in it.

She quickly came up with almost a dozen certainties, (*not mere assumptions*, she assured herself) about her condition. It was so easy to be brutally honest with herself. She tidily wrote her list on a sheet of paper.

What I know for sure about my health CONDITION

1. My lows are caused by a character flaw.
2. I deserve to be depressed because of this character flaw.
3. I'm weak and can't handle the little lows in life like other people can.
4. Having depression is my own fault.
5. It is a problem that can be fixed by psychotherapy, if I do it for the rest of my life.
6. I got it from my father.
7. I will either grow out of having depressions, or I will grow old with them.
8. I get depressed partly because I have no coping skills like other people do.
9. I may not ever come out of a future episode.
10. I could be cured for good if I really wanted to be, if I worked hard enough, but I'm just too lazy to do that.
11. If I moved to a better climate, I probably wouldn't get depressed.

Proudly, Brenda went to her next appointment, completed assignment in hand. Her shrink looked it over and put it down on his desk.

All he said was, "I'll keep this, and we'll deal with it later."

That sounded awfully strange to Brenda, and she was a bit disappointed that she didn't have the opportunity to defend her points, but she agreed to his decision.

"Now I have a list for you," he said, retrieving a single sheet of paper from his briefcase and offering it to her.

Facts about uni-polar depression

1. Uni-polar depression is believed to be caused by a chemical imbalance in the brain, to do with neurotransmitters.
2. This type of depression can be treated, but no cure has yet been found for it.
3. Uni-polar depression is called a mood disorder, which falls within the medical category of mental illness.
4. It is also called endogenous depression, meaning that it is not precipitated or caused by any particular external event(s).
5. A person with uni-polar mood disorder recovers from episodes, but the illness may remain.
6. An episode is physically over when the brain chemistry returns to normal.
7. There is no blood test to tell when blood chemistry is normal again.
8. Uni-polar depression is often successfully treated with medication and/or therapy.
9. People with uni-polar mood disorder can help themselves in their recovery from episodes.

Brenda read quickly and abruptly dropped the piece of paper on the table, as if it was a hot potato. "I won't touch this!"

"Why not?"

"It says I have a mental illness."

"It says a lot of other things as well."

"I don't care. I will never believe, let alone admit, that I have a mental illness."

"Brenda," the shrink said in his now-I'm-going-to-tell-you-something-important voice, "you have experienced bouts of depression since you were 17. They have not been a result of your not being able to deal with school, your family, your friends, or the world. They have occurred because you have a chemical imbalance in your brain. I can explain this to you if you like."

He paused briefly, then continued. "You may have inherited this illness from your father, who you say has also suffered many episodes of depression. In any case, this disorder, this illness, is not your fault, and, whether you like it or not, it is referred to as a mental illness."

Brenda felt trapped and in a panic. "No! I will not accept that label."

"Well, could you accept the label 'illness'?"

"No!" Brenda responded frantically.

How can I get out of here? I'm not sick! I don't have an illness. I just get depressed sometimes!

"I want you to think about this until our next appointment. I want you to think about the advantages of naming your 'condition' as you call it, an 'illness'."

This was the dirtiest trick he'd ever sprung on her. But, he'd given her some pretty weird and irritating assignments before, which she had carried out. And she'd been glad of it afterwards. She decided to comply.

She tackled the assignment with her usual zest. She was going to find 10 good reasons for calling her depressions an "illness," even if it killed her.

She let go of her resistance to "illness." As long as she didn't put "mental" in front of it, she was okay.

Brenda thought of other illnesses, just to get a handle on the word. Diabetes came to mind. Thinking of diabetes made it much easier for her to list her reasons, taking into account the shrink's list. She even consulted a medical dictionary for a definition of the word illness. In a short time, she came up with ten very good reasons to call her depressions an illness. She wrote them out and took them to her next appointment.

"Here they are," she said in a tone, that implied, "You asked for it; you got it."

If I call my condition an illness, then:

1. It's not my fault.
2. I don't deserve to have it: no one deserves to be ill.
3. It may have a bio-chemical or some sort of physical basis.
4. Running away from it can't cure me. In fact, I probably can't be cured at all.
5. There is a good chance it can be treated, at least with medication.
6. Therapy may be able to help.
7. Maybe there are support groups for depressed people; there seem to be for so many other illnesses.
8. For me this illness is chronic, repeating.
9. I've good reason to be outraged, disappointed, and sad because I waste so much time being ill.
10. This illness is confined to my body. It doesn't run rampant through my heart and soul, even though it may show in my behavior and in my feelings about myself.

The shrink read the points carefully. "Very good, Brenda. Now, let me ask you one more thing."

Brenda thought, *As if I have a choice,* but said, "Like what?"

"You seem comfortable with the word illness now, am I right?"

"Mostly."

"Well, why don't we put the word mental in front of it? Because that is the case, you know."

"No way. Being mentally ill means I'm nuts, that I belong in the loonie bin, that I can't get along in the world. And, besides, I've never even been in the hospital."

"That's the stigma attached to the term mental illness, not the fact. Besides, I'm not suggesting that you tell everyone you have a mental illness, just that you recognize it yourself. If you do, you'll be able to deal with it straight on, rather than treating it as something vague and unclear. As you've indicated, there is a similarity between depression and diabetes: in both cases people often require medication to correct an imbalance. But the difference with depression is that episodes are accompanied by mental manifestations that have to be contended with, such as," he paused, "your Dark Pit, mental exhaustion, confusion, absent-mindedness, diminished intellectual capability, lowered self-esteem." He paused again. "Is this not true?"

Damn it, Brenda thought, *he's right.* "I still don't like it."

"I know. And you don't have to like it. But if you accept it, you can find resources out in the world that can support you." He hesitated. "You wouldn't choose to read a book with the words 'mental illness' in the title, would you?"

"No, I certainly wouldn't."

"That's a pity, because there is a very fine book called 'Grieving Mental Illness,' and I highly recommend that you read it."

Brenda left the appointment angrily. *I hate that man,* she said to herself.

She contemplated that conversation for a week. She was, in turn, angry and curious. Today, her curiosity got the better of her. So she quietly went into her bedroom, locked the door, and took out her journal. She tentatively wrote in small, almost indiscernible letters, "I have a mental illness."

Oh, God, I can't stand it!

She stroked through the words so thoroughly that even she, at some future date, wouldn't be able to tell what she had written. She was sorely tempted to slam her journal shut. She took a deep breath.

But this is my own assignment. I am not going to give in.

Again she wrote in small letters, "I have a mental illness." This time she didn't strike it out the instant she had written it.

Whatever it is, I certainly don't deserve it. Thank heavens no one can see me write this. She looked around to make sure.

Again she wrote, "I have a mental illness."

Well, I have an illness. I'll admit that much. Her words were legible this time.

Again she wrote, "I have a mental illness."

This is such a stupid exercise, and *I'm doing it of my own free will. I am crazy!* She laughed to herself.

Again she wrote, "I have a mental illness."

I understand by mental that my illness affects my feelings, my intellect, and my self-esteem. She breathed a bit easier and reviewed her five statements, which looked increasingly like they had been written in her own handwriting.

Again she wrote, "I have a mental illness."

This is a pretty idiotic thing to do. Why am I doing it anyway? Oh yeah. Because I'm stubborn, and I promised myself I would. It's still stupid.

Again she wrote, "I have a mental illness."

Well, I may as well settle in with this, because I'm going to write this acknowledgment, this admission, until I feel comfortable with it.

Again she wrote, "I have a mental illness."

I wonder whether that book he mentioned is any good. 'Grieving Mental Illness,' wasn't it? Maybe I'll see if it's at the library.

Again she wrote, "I have a mental illness."

Well, I can say that to myself, but I don't have to admit it to anyone else. She looked around again to make certain no one could see her.

Again she wrote, "I have a mental illness."

The stigma of "mental illness" is horrible. It's unfair. But that's how a mood disorder is defined medically; that's how it's viewed in literature, in research. Maybe I could accept it in those contexts. It may even be to my advantage to do so. But I still hate the stigma.

She was a little bit taken aback by her rising resentment of the stigma attached to the term and with her increasing comfort with the repeated statement.

How can I be having these opposite feelings at the same time?

By the time she'd written her statement forty times, Brenda was fairly comfortable with it.

Certainly not fully comfortable. I still don't want to discuss it. Not even with Mom. But I understand the meaning of my illness a lot better now. That's such a relief, such a good place to start from

187

tomorrow, she tells herself as she caps her pen and puts her journal away in its usual safe place.

Brenda sighs. She is very pleased with herself.

Imagine

Have you ever tried to imagine what your life would be like—would have been like—if you didn't have a mood disorder? I have, and I suspect you have too.

I can't imagine being a 5'2" male Chinese immigrant to Canada who hasn't learned the English language, when I am a 5'9" female whose family has been Canadian for three generations and who doesn't know one word in any other language. You can't imagine what it is like to be, as Helen Keller was, blind and deaf throughout life, unless you are. We can pretend to have their characteristics perhaps for an hour or a day, but we cannot in all honesty imagine being these people.

So, why do we try to imagine life without a mood disorder?

I believe that we do this because curiosity in any human being is a natural, usually healthy, activity. Where would we be if we didn't imagine at all in our lives? There may be something to be gained through imagining many sorts of things—for you and me, a life without a mood disorder. It is certainly understandable, however, that one might hesitate to venture down that wondering path, which can so easily become fruitless and frustrating.

But it needn't be so.

Recently I dared to ask myself how much time I have spent going into, being in, and coming out of depressive episodes. I was shocked and dismayed when I summed up the months and months—too many months.

After a short but cathartic cry, I asked myself, "What could and would I have done with my life had it been otherwise?" Merely asking the question frightened me, as I thought I might conclude that my life, so marked with black holes, has been a terrible waste.

Afraid or not, I had to face that question and the more specific one, "What career might I otherwise have chosen?"

For the first time in my life, I allowed myself to fully consider and honestly answer the question.

I would have continued my education, entering a cross-disciplinary program including language, mathematics, and spirituality. By now I would probably be a professor with tenure at a small university. I would have written a book or two and would have a comfortable pension to look forward to.

It seemed only fair to ask myself, after this make believe, "What have I done with what I've been given?" Yes, life has given us this disorder. We have come by it honestly, many of us through family genes. We haven't "made up" our illness for some perverse or compensatory reason.

In terms of my own real career, I have taken on meaningful work and have become respected in my field. I have carved out an authentic life style and have nurtured a loving heart partnership. And I am writing about mood disorders, which is one thing I have always wanted to do.

The short answer to "What have I done...?" is "The best I could do," and I am doing my best now within the existing parameters of self-understanding, evolving medications, compassionate friends and family, and competent medical care.

In order to live at peace with myself and to be able to say, "This has been, and is, a worthwhile life," I have shielded myself from anticipated intense disappointment by not asking, "What could I have done?" Shielding myself from this pain has, until now, been permissible, possibly even advisable.

My life couldn't have been different back then. I had not lost valuable opportunities. I had merely missed out on impossibilities. I realize that I cannot change the past.

Now, having asked and answered the "back then" question, I can quite honestly say, "This has been my life. This is my life. And it *is* worthwhile."

The most I, or anyone, can do today is live fully in the present. The future for those of us with mood disorders looks brighter than ever before. Medical science is progressing, if slower than we'd like, and there will, no doubt, be better medications around the corner. On the personal front, I will continue with the excellent ongoing medical care I have carefully chosen and maintained, and I will continue to seek and apply new techniques of self-care.

Now instead of asking myself, "What if I didn't have this disorder?", I ask, "What more can I do, given that I have it?" This one question breaks down into several questions: "What more can

I do for myself, and for others with mood disorders and for people with other disorders and for the larger community around me?"

From what I have seen and heard at support group meetings, other people who recognize that they have a mood disorder are asking similar questions. The answers are many and diverse. Here are a few of mine:

- By doing the best for myself, I can be a functioning and contributing member of society, and not a heavy weight on the medical system; I can confront this immense challenge in my life and gain strength.
- By helping others with the illness, I can perhaps make a positive difference in their bumpy journeys.
- By my example and by communicating with them, I can show people with other disorders that we share much in our separate struggles to reach and maintain good mental health.
- By telling my stories to others in the community around me, I can give people the opportunity to not feel sorry for me but to feel compassion for me and to gain an understanding of mental unwellness; I can give them a chance to participate more meaningfully in my life by opening myself to them, and I can give myself the opportunity to participate more meaningfully in their lives as well.

Clearly, there is benefit all around.

Imagine that!

Section 4:

Since You Asked

There and Back

What's it like?" Emma asked quietly, shyly, as if the question had to do with sex, or life in jail, or the death of a child. In fact, she was asking Jess what it's like to experience an episode of depression.

Jess is an expert on the topic of episodes. She's gone through a dozen or so in her life. Too many, too long, too much.

She would usually reply to the what's-it-like question very prosaically. She couldn't tell whether the questioner was truly interested, feigning interest, or just snoopy, so she'd say something like, "Oh, it's awful: it's emotionally painful, and it's terribly exhausting." Then she would change the subject.

But Jess knew Emma well enough to know that she was sincere. It was clear that she sympathized, that the backdrop of her question was, "I wonder what I could do to help at those times."

So, this time, with Emma, whom she trusted, and with whom she had shared other personal concerns, Jess wanted to be more specific. She wanted to offer her friend an understanding of the experience, or as much of an understanding as one on the outside could possibly have. But she couldn't, on the spot, find the words to do it justice.

Despite her many episodes, she had never tried to put the experience into words, even to herself. When she was in an episode, she couldn't put words to anything, let alone describe the hell she was going through. And when she was well, she didn't like to think about being ill. In fact, she could barely relate to the illness. It seemed like an unbelievable story of someone else's life. Certainly not hers.

This made her feel that her life was discontinuous: she was either "here" (well) or "there" (ill). She wondered if "normal" people experienced that sort of discontinuity. Would recurring depression compare to any other illness in that respect: cancer, diabetes, multiple sclerosis...? Would an epileptic or an asthmatic have to struggle as she does towards continuity?

Her mind returned to Emma's question, "I'd really like to answer that, but to be honest, I don't know how. Let me think about it for a bit."

"Sure," Emma replied, puzzled by her friend's hesitation.

Jess was usually very good at explaining things on the spot. Just last week, she had talked about her para-gliding experience. At the end of the story, Emma felt she'd been along for the ride.

Ah, well, she thought, *I can wait for this one.*

Over the next few days, Jess dared to look at those unhappy periods of her life—the recurring bouts of depression so tidily labeled "episodes."

That Place is how she refers to the place where she seems to exist during the painful times, That Place being the least emotional name she can find for it. By merely thinking about that dark and terrible place, she is afraid she might bring the Dark Presence—the inner voice that torments her during episodes—to the fore again. She takes some of the sting out of that nasty entity by shortening it to DP.

Jess promised herself that she would persevere with any emotional pain she suffered in her search for the right words to describe her episodes.

It's time to do more than just name That Place. I need to focus on it, to even risk touching it briefly. It might be the only way to get to the heart of the matter. That's scary. But if I do it, I might learn something new—if, that is, I can keep myself at a safe distance where I can't be sucked in. I'll need to be ready to run the other direction at any moment.

Yes, that's her usual crisis management strategy, her disaster recovery route. *Not very dignified, but it'll probably work.*

After about a week of working on the assignment, and managing to prevent herself from slipping into That Place, she felt ready to share her insights.

I mustn't overstate it or Emma won't believe me. But I mustn't depict something so painful and frightening as bland. This'll be a fine line to walk.

A few days later, Jess and Emma met for dinner at Minerva's, a restaurant they enjoyed for its quiet ambiance and great food.

196

After they were seated by the window, Jess announced that she felt able to express what an episode is like.

Before they opened their menus, she warned, "You'll have to use your imagination for this."

"No problem. I like learning that way."

After the waiter had poured them some wine, Jess took a deep breath, ready to embark, as if on a medieval journey of great consequence, and began her story.

"Imagine your life as a walk along a path."

A safe start. So many people these days see life as a journey.

"You travel up and down hills, around bends, on rough gravel and smooth pavement. There are days and nights corresponding to your light and dark times. These represent periods of time going smoothly and well, and other periods of crisis, pain, and estrangement."

"Right."

"People with recurring depression experience an additional variety of these days and nights."

"Okay."

"So, imagine people who experience recurring depressions as having something special that occurs for them on this path now and again. And imagine the place where this special thing occurs as a room with four walls, a ceiling and a floor, and no apparent doors or windows. It's like a 10 foot box which is just plunked in front of them at any time, whether they are on the top of a hill at noon or quietly watching the sun set or riding rough waves. Now, imagine that you are one of these people, and you are now facing one of these boxes, one of these rooms."

"Alright." Emma breathed deeply, preparing herself for she didn't know what. She took a good big sip of wine.

"You look closely at this box. It's so different from anything else you've met along the path, so out of place. And yet you remember facing it before, having to deal with it before.

"You remember it as a deeply dark and dreadful place, one which you would certainly not choose to enter.

"It moves closer and closer to you, taunting you, crowding you, threatening you, and you begin to panic.

197

"Now, sometimes you can stop its motion towards you, and even make it back off or disappear. Other times, it keeps moving towards you gradually, slowly, unavoidably. And at still other times you feel yourself shoved into it from behind. In any event, you enter it most unwillingly."

"Okay, okay," said Emma, nervously. "I'm with you so far."

"So, in this box, this room, which you call That Place, all you see is blackness. You don't know where the room ends, because you can't see the walls. You hardly know which way is up, let alone the direction in which you are meant to go. You turn around and become totally disoriented. You realize you're trapped, absolutely alone, with no guarantees, indeed no hope, of getting out soon. And you know, from experience, that panic does you no good. But you panic nonetheless. It's a knee-jerk reaction."

"I'm not enjoying That Place." Emma shuddered.

"Let's take a bit of a break," Jess offered. "Well timed! Here's our food."

After they had eaten in reflective silence for a while, Jess continued.

"Now, the room, That Place, is bitterly cold. A terrible wind is howling, and you are terrified. You feel your own inner light dimming.

"After being here for only a short time, you begin to believe that you have always lived here. There is no outside of this room. There are no pathways within or without. There is only blackness and bleakness, aloneness and loneliness."

As if to give credence to her story, dusk was settling outside, the day's light fading.

"Now a stereo is turned on nearby. There is the ominous sound of drumming. You hear a voice. It starts speaking softly and you strain to hear. With the increasing volume of the voice, you are soon shocked to recognize it as your very own voice, talking, then yelling terrible, contemptuous things at you. 'You're a lousy, lazy, useless blob.' The voice is relentless in its cruelty. You feel more and more trapped. You think you will die here. 'There's no way out of this,' the voice yells. 'You're going to be in this hell forever, just as you deserve. You're so useless. You're nothing. You're nothing to anybody. Shame on you for taking up valuable space!' You cover your ears with your hands, but it doesn't help. The voice only gets louder. You now realize that what you are hearing is the voice of the Dark Presence."

"The Dark Presence?"

Jess topped up both their wine glasses as she explained the horrible, invisible phantom that torments and mocks her incessantly when she's depressed.

"You try to bargain with the Dark Presence. But it carries on shouting at you, ignoring all your pitiful pleas. After a while, you're worn out, defenseless. Soon you believe everything it says.

"You have to get away from this hell, so you decide to sleep, but you can't close your eyes. After what seems an eternity, you finally drop off, but awaken three hours later in the middle of a nightmare. The stereo continues to blast its profanities and insults at you. You cry, you scream, you run around hoping to find a door out of this hell. There isn't one." She paused, hoping that she wasn't being too graphic.

Well, that's exactly what it feels like, she assured herself.

"You try to recall inspirational words you have tucked away in your notebook, but, of course, you don't have your notebook with you. All you can manage to retrieve from some dark corner of your brain is the expression, 'This too will pass.' You know that this is a complete lie. The Dark Presence is mocking you."

She paused again and looked at an incredulous Emma, who had stopped eating and drinking.

"You think I'm exaggerating, don't you?"

"It does sound a bit extreme."

"It is extreme. That's the nature of the illness."

"Well, it sounds absolutely dreadful, but I do believe you, Jess." Emma squirmed a bit in her chair, quietly hoping that she wouldn't have to hear more. But Jess ignored her friend's discomfort.

"Finally, after a few weeks or months of this agony, this self-torment, you fall to your knees, exhausted. You feel as though you've been reduced to nothing. Your self has left, and any light within you has been extinguished. And still the voice, <u>your</u> voice, yells at you, screams at you."

"Okay, okay!" Emma almost shouted. "I really do get it. Can we stop this now please?"

"All right, Emma," Jess replied, lowering her voice, and pausing as the waiter cleared the table.

"Several months after being there, with nothing improving, when you've given up on being rescued or rescuing yourself, one day you see a very dim shaft of light. It seems far away, and you can't tell whether its source is in That Place or not. That doesn't matter. It <u>is</u> light. You stand up and rush towards it, desperately. You try to grab it. It disappears. It's pitch dark again. Then the light returns a few more times, and you grab for it again and again. It always evades you.

"Finally, wisely, you decide on another strategy. The next time the light appears, you'll follow it, rather than try to seize it. So the next time, you walk, and you finally come close to it. It backs off. You are really frustrated. But you keep your eye on it.

"After a very long while, the light settles on one spot, showing you the direction you need to take. You dare to think that maybe there <u>is</u> a way out of here. You walk and walk, following the silent promise, wondering how far you will have to go. Finally, you see a faint outline of a window." She stopped to make sure Emma was still with her.

Emma looked as if she'd been running.

Jess changed the subject abruptly. "How about dessert?"

"No, thanks. Please continue." Emma wanted to be out of That Place as soon as possible and waited anxiously as Jess ordered coffee.

"At this point, you sense your own inner light beginning to warm up and shine once again and you think, 'Thank God, my spirit hasn't died after all!' You are immensely relieved. With these two lights—one from within, one from without—you dare to think that maybe this ordeal will be over soon.

"You begin to see outlines of more windows. You walk slowly towards one of them, keeping a constant eye on it, as if that will prevent it from disappearing. As you get closer, you can see, through the window, that there is real life out there, other people, other things going on. It looks strange, unfamiliar, as if you'd been transported to a foreign country.

"You realize that the hell you've experienced for months is, in fact, an episode of your illness and has not been of your own making. Your shame starts to lift; your guilt eases. Good feelings about yourself gradually return, not to mention your 'proper' imagination. The Dark Presence has gone."

"Thank God!" Emma exclaimed.

Jess gave Emma a moment to catch up.

"There's more, Emma. But the next part won't be so painful."

"Thank you very much!"

"Your history of recurring depressions, your visits to the hell of That Place, has taught you that trying to perceive continuity in your life is very important, if often impossible.

"You know that climbing out through a window and slamming it behind you is not the best action. Your recent experience in That Place has been part of your life, not apart from it. It's tempting to see it as an interruption or an aberration, but it has been your life for all those months.

"As horrible as the hell was, you want to integrate the experience into your larger, longer, life. You gather all your returning resources, wanting to create a remembrance of this experience, to celebrate the light returning and the appearance of the windows. When you were coming out of your last episode, you drew a picture of a huge sun. This time, words seem like the best way to express how you feel. After a few awkward attempts, you come up with a poem that expresses your relief, your pleasure, your gratitude that you can now leave That Place."

Jess reached into her pocket, retrieved a carefully folded piece of paper, and gave it to Emma.

"Your poem may go something like this. I wrote it after a recent episode. I don't really fancy myself a poet, but writing verse has helped me to get through many depressions."

Emma read it silently, as Jess sipped on her coffee.

A glimmer, a shimmer of unmistakable light,
Relief from the presence of this necessary night.

Light through the windows, windows easing the pain,
A cleansing, a clearing brought here by the rain.

This room full of windows, which open and close,
Bringing fresh air and promise to the blossoming rose.

This room full of feelings, some sadness, some sorrow,
But room for the upswing of some soon tomorrow.

There's much to be learned here at this time of mourning,
When the sun gets eclipsed with no prior warning.

For now, I will stay here and do what I must
To nurture the healing, encourage new trust.

Yes, this is my home in which I will stay
Until I am ready to venture away

Through some open window (which one I can't say)
But for sure it will lead me to the brightness of day.

When she had finished reading, Emma put the paper down.
"I call it *In Praise of Windows* because it celebrates, affirms."
Jess paused to remember how she had felt when she composed this poem. There was a sense of completion, of new freedom, indeed new life at the time. She had those very same feelings now too.

"You're pleased with your effort," she said, carrying on with her story. "Yes, it expresses how you feel. You re-read it, fold it up, put it in your pocket to take with you.

"Now you must choose a window to climb through. You do so, hoping that by climbing through this one you will find yourself near to where you were when this episode began. But then, you can hardly remember where you were those many weeks or months ago.

"As you step onto real earth again, you are almost blinded by the light of day. You try to get your bearings, but you aren't in the same place you were in before your journey was so agonizingly interrupted. You have to start again from a new place. But, that's okay.

"Finally, you are at home on your path. You look around, reconnect with friends, and celebrate your return. Now you are ready for the next hill, the next bend in the road."

"Thank heavens." Emma was looking quite exhausted by now, but she was also visibly relieved.

"You have a pretty good idea that you'll encounter That Place again, but here and now is your healthy life. You know there's no use worrying about next time. You walk along.

"Well, that's one way of looking at an episode," Jess said, as she finished her coffee. "Could I offer you a few other ways?"

"Absolutely not! At least not right now, thank you very much. But thanks for telling me what it's like. I almost feel as if I've been there and back myself!"

"Great! That was my intention."

Jess relaxed her now very weary body and mind. She had successfully completed the task she had set herself.

Jess and Emma paid the bill and walked out into the fresh evening air.

Dare to Ask

If you know that I sky-dive for recreation, and if you are interested in understanding something of the sport, you may want to ask me questions about it, questions such as: Why do you do it? What does it feel like to be in mid-air? Don't you worry about your parachute not opening?

If you ask me these questions, I will be willing, indeed eager, to answer them. I will be pleased that you are interested enough to ask.

As I answer your questions, you may imagine sky-diving yourself, or you may compare it to some activity you do, or have done, that may be similar, for instance, jumping from a diving board into a swimming pool.

If you know that I experience recurring bouts of depression, and if you are interested in understanding me and my illness better, you may want to ask me questions about it.

If you ask me questions about my illness, I will most likely be pleased that you are interested enough to ask.

But you may feel reticent about approaching me with your questions. This is natural.

Asking a person about any illness is a delicate matter, much more so than asking about sky-diving, and could be interpreted as an invasion of privacy.

You may fear that your questions, or my reflections on my illness, will trigger an episode, or that you will be vulnerable to depression if you get too close to me. And, if, or as, I answer your questions, you may remember times when you've felt low and try to compare your feelings with mine.

If you decide that you will dare to ask, you might consider examining your own motives and the depth of your interest.

If your interest is of a superficial, passing nature, perhaps some pamphlets from your local Mental Health or Mood Disorders Association would satisfy your curiosity.

Even assuming that your interest arises from a deeper, more abiding concern, there are a number of things that you should think about.

Predicting anyone's receptivity at any time to highly personal questions is chancy at best. It is at times very difficult for me to find the words to express my thoughts and feelings. And at times I simply do not want to talk.

You could ask me directly if I am able and willing to tell you about my illness, or you could take the roundabout route and ask my partner or best friend for advice on whether and how to approach me with your request for information.

Whichever route you choose, you must approach carefully. Though you don't yet know what my responses will be, it is best to be prepared to spend as much time as it takes for me to say what I have to say.

If I am willing to talk, you might explain that if there are aspects of my illness that I don't wish to discuss, you will respect the limitations. And it would be wise to add, "I'll understand if you begin to feel uncomfortable and want to stop at any time." I hope I would remember to say the same to you, as sometimes you, too, may feel vulnerable talking about this topic, and, if you wish, we should stop discussing it when you feel at all nervous or insecure.

Key your questions to what you perceive my mental state to be at the time. If my mood is on a downward slope, or if I am just beginning to emerge from an episode, it's best to ask me relatively elementary questions. I probably won't have the energy or thinking power to respond to complex philosophical queries at that time. Save your more probing questions for when I am in good mental health.

And finally, please recognize and remember that my answers are not universal. They apply to me. I can speak only for myself. If you apply what I say to someone else about whom you are concerned, you do so at great risk to you both.

Whether I answer all, or some, or—if our timing is bad—none of your questions, be assured I will most likely be pleased that you are interested enough to ask. Your sitting with me and asking about me and listening to me shows me that you care and helps me to feel less isolated.

Below are several questions you may want to ask someone you know who experiences recurring depression.

Easiest questions:

- How did you get this illness? Why you and not me?
- Are you taking medication? Do you think it does you any good? Do you experience side effects? Are there constraints? (For instance, can you drink alcohol?)
- Do you meet with a psychiatrist regularly? If so, do you think it helps?
- Have you tried a variety of therapies for your illness, for instance, orthodox Western medicine, homeopathy, special diet, body work, etc.?
- How often do you have episodes, and how long do they usually last? Do you have an idea when you will have your next one?
- Are you able to anticipate how long it will take you to recover from an episode?
- Do you feel the same depth of pain each time?
- Could talking about it when you are well make you vulnerable to slipping into an episode?
- Could external factors, such as money, marital, or business problems cause you to slip?
- Do you think the loss of a friendship, a loved one, or a job could precipitate an episode?
- Does your family know about your illness? People at work? What was it like telling them?
- How does your family (parents, siblings, partner, children) respond to your illness?
- How do you handle a situation where a person minimizes your illness (for instance, says, "We all get the blues now and then," or, "You'll grow out of it")?

Delicate questions:

- What's the worst aspect of an episode for you?
- Have you ever been hospitalized for depression?

- Do you think that you will have depressive episodes for the rest of your life?
- Are you sometimes afraid you will never come out of an episode?
- Do you fear that you will die while you are in an episode?
- Should people with debilitating episodes have children?
- Do medications affect sex drive or fertility?
- Do depressive episodes affect sex drive?

Questions on ongoing living with recurring depression:

- Do you feel bitter about having the illness? Do you think that life isn't fair?
- Do you feel you have lost valuable and productive time because of your episodes?
- Why bother with a career and other goals with all the interruptions episodes bring?
- What carries you through an episode?
- What prevents you from giving in or giving up during long episodes?
- What makes your life worth living if you are quite certain that you will suffer deep depressions repeatedly in the future?

Questions concerning a supporter's involvement:

- My partner has recurring depression. What does this mean to me?
- How can I find out more about this illness?
- Might I get depressed by being around you a lot when you are depressed?
- How can I help?

Ultimate questions:
- Have you ever thought of committing suicide? If so, how did you think you would do it?
- If you've thought about committing suicide but have not tried to, what stopped you?
- Have you ever tried to commit suicide? What happened?

The above questions may lead you to more questions concerning recurring depression.

You will find some of my responses to these questions in the articles and stories of this book.

If you have more questions or are hesitant to ask your friend or loved one about recurring depression, refer to the Suggested Reading List at the end of this book or ask your own doctor.

Asking About the Worst

Devon hadn't had the nerve to ask his friend Andrew whether he'd ever attempted to commit suicide. He couldn't even bring himself to ask whether he'd ever thought about it.

It's not morbid curiosity, he'd assured himself. *It's genuine concern, and I'd really like to be as supportive as I possibly can.*

Devon had no idea how Andrew would respond to such personal questions. They'd been friends for about five years. They'd talked a bit about Andrew's depressions but no deep stuff. The suicide issue was in danger of becoming an obsession to Devon, and he knew that if he let it go that far without dealing with it, he might start drawing away from Andrew.

I can't let that happen. I've just got to ask.

Easier said than done. Not that Andrew was overly sensitive about talking about his mood disorder.

He always sounds so matter of fact when he says anything about his depressions. He's so rational about it all. And thank heavens he doesn't talk about it incessantly. I couldn't take that.

Andrew had explained to Devon that it doesn't help to be emotional when he talks about his illness.

"Besides, I can't really feel the desperation, the agony of a low when I'm well, even when I'm talking about it. It's like being on the other side of a gigantic stone wall."

Devon was getting impatient with himself. *So, why don't I just come out and ask him? Am I afraid that I won't be able to handle the response? Hmm... Maybe I am. Am I afraid he'll tell me to mind my own business? No, I don't think so. Am I afraid my questions might bring on an episode? I don't think so, but I don't really know. Maybe it's just too risky.*

Devon was driving himself nuts with these worries.

Maybe when the time seems right, I could lead up to it gradually, test the waters. I've got to get rid of my worries or confirm them. No more excuses!

* * *

211

Last weekend the two friends went hiking. About half way along the trail, they found a fallen tree and decided to sit down and have a drink.

The time is now, Devon thought, and before he could think any more about it, he said, "Andrew, I've been wondering about some personal aspects of your illness."

"Yeah, like what?"

"Well, first of all, do you mind talking about it now?"

"Not at all."

"I was afraid that talking about really painful stuff might throw you into an episode, or maybe it's just too private for you to talk about."

"No, it's fine. Thanks anyway. Actually, it's a relief to be asked personal questions. Most people don't ask. When I do talk, I always learn something, get new insights. I welcome it like a fresh breeze on a hot day." He paused. "But if I go on and on and it gets to be too much for you, ask me to stop. Okay?"

"That's a deal. And I'll stop you if I think it's getting to be hard on you too."

"Good idea."

Andrew waited silently, albeit a bit nervously, for the first question, and Devon sensed his nervousness.

"Do you need time to think it over?"

"No. It's okay. I just have to make sure I'm grounded—you know, balanced—to talk about it."

"Yeah, I think I know what you mean."

In a few minutes Andrew was ready for whatever Devon wanted to ask him.

"Okay. Well... I'm wondering what your worst fears are about your illness." Devon blurted it out, so he wouldn't trip up in the middle of the sentence and chicken out.

"Mmm... I've never been asked exactly that before. But I've thought enough about it." Another pause. "Actually, I have two immense fears... and I couldn't tell you which is worst. That doesn't matter, of course...." Andrew trailed off, then promptly got back on track. "One is that I might go insane—go mad—when the torment is unbearable... that I'll withdraw so much from everyone and

212

everything, that I'll be committed to—I hate that term—a mental hospital, the loonie bin as some like to call it." He gave Devon a moment to digest that.

"The other is that I might kill myself some day during an episode because there's absolutely no way I can stand the agony, the torture, anymore." Andrew shivered for a moment, then added, "So, there you are. The bottom line."

"Whew!"

Knowing that Devon would want more than the short answer, Andrew continued, "About going insane.... My mother was put in a mental hospital when I was about 15. She'd been acting really weird at home. That was scary. It was dreadful. The psychiatrist said that there was no option. She might kill herself.

"We visited her at the mental hospital a few times. It was awful. One locked door after another, people with vacant stares rocking in their chairs. It was downright frightening. I could be one of those people sometime." Andrew looked somber, but continued. "I'm afraid of being put away like that some day. That terrifies me. I think being put in a straight jacket and doped up and locked up would be more humiliating than being dead."

He quickly realized the irony in his statement. *Humour's good,* he sighed. It wasn't lost on Devon either. They both smiled weakly.

"The going insane fear is with me all the time, whether I'm well or ill. It's like someone skulking behind me, ready to pounce when I'm most vulnerable. I've talked about it with my therapist over the years. I'm less afraid than I used to be. But there aren't any guarantees that I won't go the way of Mom. It might be genetic, you know."

Devon didn't know what to say, so said nothing.

"Want more about that one?"

"No. No thanks. That's enough of that for now. Let's walk. Can we walk and talk?"

For Devon it was definitely time to move on. *This is scary stuff. I can't imagine Andrew being locked up.*

They walked along in silence for some time. "How about your second fear?" Devon asked, still unable to mouth the "s" word.

"Ah, yes. About killing myself... I fear the suicide impulse only when I'm deeply depressed. In fact, it's hard to believe, right this minute, when I'm in really good mental health, that it is, or ever has been, a concern. But I do believe it. I know it to be true. I know it's a life-threatening concern when I am acutely depressed."

Andrew noticed Devon's quizzical expression. "What I mean is, I don't put myself down for having the impulse, and I know I have to deal very seriously with it when it appears. If I didn't respect it, take it seriously, I'm sure I would've done myself in by now."

Devon looked for a comparison in his own life. *If I didn't take drinking and driving seriously, I probably wouldn't be here either.*

"Sometimes when I'm really in despair, when I feel hopeless and helpless, I feel like I'm floating alone, completely alone, in cold, black darkness at the periphery of the universe. The 'I' of me feels smaller than a sesame seed, almost obliterated. I don't have any soul left. My mind screams out that I am less than useless. Nothing matters. I feel so lonely, so cut off, so distant from everything and everybody.

"At the time, I can't see any solution to the situation. I can't stand the agony anymore. I have to stop the screaming inside. I feel totally, utterly defeated. I have to get out of where I am, out of my body, and there's no way to do that and stay in this world.

"That's when suicidal thoughts enter my mind. They're not something I choose. I don't want them. But soon they flood right in. Sometimes they take over, and I can't think of anything other than suicide. Killing myself is the only way out.

"In a way, this is comforting to me, because I realize I can escape this torment." Andrew took a deep breath. "Living isn't possible. I've just gone beyond."

"Gone beyond? I don't quite get that."

"I know. It's hard to explain, but I'll try if you want."

"Please do. I'd like to understand it."

"I've gone beyond hope, beyond caring, and even beyond feeling. I become rational, if only to myself. Killing myself becomes a project, the most important project I have ever undertaken. I need to plan it thoroughly and execute it well. I even get excited about it." Andrew stopped. He could hardly believe what he was saying.

But it's the truth. That is what it's like.

Devon was becoming concerned about Andrew's increasing momentum and excitement. He hesitated. *Should I stop him? No, maybe it's better to get it all out.*

"So, have you... have you ever tried it?"

"No. No I haven't." Andrew returned to the present. "Got close a couple of times. The first time I didn't do it because I knew it would hurt my family too much. Even though I couldn't stand living inside this body, there was still something in me that realized they cared for me. That stopped me the first time.

"By the time I was suicidal again, about eight years later, I'd decided that my parents and sister could look after themselves if I killed myself. So I didn't have that to fall back on.

"But fortunately there was a new safeguard. This time I was faced with the prospect of hell. I couldn't convince myself there isn't a hell—and if I killed myself, hell is exactly where I would end up. Eternity is a very long time to be in scorching flames. I couldn't face that. So I endured, somehow, until my living hell was over.

"After I got over that crisis, my therapist said to me one day, 'Suicide is a permanent solution to a temporary problem, you know.' That really stuck with me. I was experienced enough with depression and suicidal thoughts by then that I knew I would at some time, some distant time, come out of each of my episodes if I hung in long enough. I became stubborn.

"By that time I'd also realized that life is really quite good during the times when I'm well, and that there are things I want to accomplish in my life.

"It all seems to boil down to, 'This too will pass.' I hate it when someone else says that to me—I hate it sometimes when I say it to myself—but it does work for me, within me."

Andrew stopped. He was exhausted, emotionally wiped. But it was good to get all this out, to put it into the air. He felt a lightness, an enormous relief.

"That's all I can do for now. Is that okay?"

"Yes. I get the picture, Andrew. I do. Yes, let's stop. Thank you. Thank you for doing this."

"It's been good for me. I really think it has. So, you're welcome, and thanks for asking."

They completed their hike in silence, in a satisfied silence.

Appendices

Special Pieces for Supporters

I hope that all the stories and articles in this book will be of interest and value to all readers. However, many of them will be of special relevance to friends, families, and supporters of people who experience recurring depression. They are:

Suggested Reading List

There are many valuable books on the market regarding depression. Several of them are listed in alphabetic sequence by author below. Some entries include a brief description of the gist of the book.

Bergen, Marja, *Riding the Roller Coaster: Living with Mood Disorders.* (Kelowna, BC: Northstone Publishing, 1999).
This is a good handbook for people who experience either bi-polar or uni-polar depression. It offers very useful suggestions, insight, and encouragement.

Health Journeys, Healthy Journeys for People with Depression. (John H Wiley and Sons)

Jamison, Kay Redfield, *An Unquiet Mind.* (NY: Random House, 1995).
An excellent well-rounded autobiography. Jamison has manic-depression. It would be useful for readers to understand this other form of mood disorder.
The book shows the importance of loving support; medication and therapy; the author uses powerful language and images.

Lafond, Virginia, *Grieving Mental Illness: A Guide for Patients and their Caregivers,* (Toronto: University of Toronto Press, 1994).
A wonderful guide for many people, and certainly those who experience recurring depression. It is fact-based, and written essentially in essay style.

Manning, Martha, *Undercurrents: A Therapist's Reckoning with Her Own Depression.*
A personal journal of recurring depression written with candor, wit and humour; Manning addresses the importance spiritual life; she explains her experience with ECT.

Morrison , M. Robert and Robert F. Stamps, *DSM-IV Internet Companion.* **(**W.W. Norton and Company, 1998)
A complete guide to over 1500 web sites offering information on mental illness, keyed to the DSM-IV.

Pinsky, Drew (ed.), *Restoring Intimacy: The Patient's Guide to Maintaining Relationships during Depression.* (Chicago: National Depressive and Manic-Depressive Association, 1999).
This book gives broad, useful suggestions on how to cope with destructive symptoms of depression such as negativity, self-degradation, unwillingness to cooperate, etc.

Styron, William, *Darkness Visible: A Memoir of Madness.* (NY: Random House, 1990).
A brilliant book on a writer's reflections on his mid-life descent into deep depression. It describes the author's depressive episode in detail, but does not offer insight into how to cope with it.

Thompson Tracy, *The Beast: Reckoning with Depression.* (NY: Putnam's Sons, 1995).
An autobiography of a woman's chronic depression; use of Prozac.

Thorne, Julia, and Rothstein, Larry, *You are Not Alone: Words of Experience and Hope for the Journey through Depression.* (NY: HarperPerennial, 1993).

Wilson, Virginia S., *Mental Illness: Survival and Beyond.* (BC: Trafford Publishing, 1998).
This concise but informative little book discusses what it is like to be hospitalized for a mental illness.

Useful Internet Resources

The internet offers thousands of websites of interest to people who want more information about mood disorders in general, and recurring depression in particular.

There is great value in browsing for information on websites. However, it can be disconcerting to do so with the huge number of sites. As well, sites can be removed at a moment's notice by the sponsors.

New websites (like new books in print) appear on a regular basis, so look for relevant new websites every few months.

One website I have found of particular value is the one whose address is:

www. mentalhealth.com.

This site, called *Internet Mental Health,* is extremely comprehensive, and has links to dozens of other useful web sites. Click on "Internet Links" then "Mood Disorders" to get a list of the referenced sites. From many of these sites you may even join discussion groups. If you have your own home computer, you can find out a great deal about depression. However, don't let the Internet be a substitute for getting proper medical or psychological attention..

To access information about recurring depression from the Internet Mental Health Home page, click on "Disorders," then "Major Depressive Disorder." From this page, you can access information on the description, symptoms, diagnosis, and treatment of recurring depression.

In addition you may see what research has been done recently concerning the illness, read numerous booklets and magazine articles on depression, including stories of personal experiences.

You may also join a Depression Web Community to get into a chat room, to post messages, and so on.

And best of all, from this web site, you can go to dozens of other websites that will offer you even more information on the illness of depression.

Other topics you will be able to read about include: types of therapy available including medication and psychotherapy; and severe depression as a biochemical illness. Read about how newer antidepressants treat the symptoms of depression more effectively, and will less troublesome side effects, than older medications. Find out ways to help a depressed person.

Information on the internet about depression is so vast that you are well advised to keep your sessions in front of the computer limited, to avoid becoming overwhelmed.

Glossary

In communicating about depressive illness, you may hear terms that you may have not heard before your introduction to the illness. Also, some day-to-day words take on new meanings. In order to converse accurately and productively about recurring depression, it is helpful to know what the various terms or words mean specifically in the context of depression.

Below I have listed and have tried to explain many terms used in this book, which you may or may not be familiar with. My descriptions and explanations are mine alone and refer to how the terms are used in this book.

These are *not* medical definitions or explanations.

For comprehensive medical definitions of words associated with recurring depression and other mood disorders, please consult a medical reference book or your doctor.

Term	Meaning given to the term in this book
Bi-polar	A mood disorder in which a person experiences cycles of mania ("highs") and depression. (Refer to the Introduction for further comments.)
Bio-chemical imbalance	One theory about the cause of recurring depression is that it is related to the activity of the neurotransmittor serotonin.
Compliance	Implies the taking of medication as prescribed. Non-compliance often leads to depressive symptoms and then to a full episode of depression.

Cure vs Treatment	There is not yet a cure for recurring depression. But, there are many treatments available including medication, various sorts of talking therapy, electro-convulsive therapy, homeopathic remedies, and so on.
Cycle	The full spectrum of moods that a person with recurring depression experiences: 1. Good mental health (wellness) 2. The descent from wellness to depression 3. Depression itself 4. Recovery to good mental health. Each of these four is a phase of the depressive cycle.
Depression causes	There may be an external precipitator for a depressive incident, or the depression may be part of a chronic illness, such as a mood disorder.
Depression Inventory Test	Many tests are available to assess a person's mental state at any given time. These tests are often administered by physicians or therapists to determine whether a person is suffering depression.
Endorphins	The brain generates these chemicals during and after the body undergoes strenuous physical activity, for instance, distance running. The effect may feel somewhat like a "high."
Episode	The period of time from when a person

begins to feel depressed until that person feels well again; that is, the descent, the actual depression, and the recovery from it.

Healing

During the recovery phase of an episode, we heal. That doesn't mean we are cured or will not have any more episodes. It means that the current episode has ended.

Illness

Recurring depression is an illness, whereas a depression caused by some external factor may not be.

Medication

Drugs may be prescribed by a physician for recurring depression. It is important to follow the directions of your physician and the prescription to achieve maximum benefit. Some people who experience recurring depression take medication all the time; others take it only during an episode of depression.

Meditation

One of many techniques that can help one feel calmer. Others include yoga, prayer, or pursuit of an art or hobby.

Mental health

Good mental health is not just the absence of illness. It is characterized by the following:
* Mentally healthy people are authentic (they are real and operate in the here and now).
* They recognize their own needs and what they need to do to satisfy them.

227

* They are open to experience.
  Even painful experiences of grief are
  part of being healthy.
* They are tolerant and accepting of
  others.

Perhaps the most crucial characteristic of
good mental health is a positive self-
concept.
This includes feeling worthwhile, and
liking oneself.

Mental illness

A category of illness used by the
medical system to do with people's
mental, as opposed to physical,
well-being. Recurring depression falls
within this category.

Mood disorder

Depression, or depression and mania, or
seasonal affective disorder.

Pill containers

Many people need to take several
medications each day, and perhaps at
several times during each day. To ensure
that you take the appropriate medication
at the appropriate times, it is a good idea
to put them into a pill box (dosette) with a
slot for each day, or get them from the
pharmacy in blister or bubble packs.

Psychotherapy

One form of treatment for depression.
It involves speaking to a mental health
professional to deal predominantly with
the emotional causes and aspects of the
depression.

Recovery

The phase in the cycle which brings one
back to good mental health. Recovery

can take a short time or several months. People in recovery often experience some good days followed by bad days until the episode is over.

Recurring depression — A type of depression that occurs over and over again during one's lifetime. (Refer to the Introduction for more details.)

Remission — The phase during which an illness is not manifested. For people with depressive illness, remission is when they are mentally well.

S.A.D. — Seasonal affective disorder, a form of mood disorder connected to the amount of sunlight each day. (See the Introduction for more.)

Support group — A gathering of persons with mood disorders, their supporters, and friends. Meetings are often conducted weekly or monthly. The facilitator is usually a person who has a mood disorder, not a medical professional.

Symptoms — Signs by which we can tell if we are at risk of entering an episode of depression. They include:
* loss of energy and interest
* diminished ability to enjoy oneself
* difficulty in concentrating
* indecisiveness
* slow or fuzzy thinking
* exaggerated feelings of sadness, hopelessness, or anxiety

* feelings of worthlessness
* recurring thoughts of death or suicide
* not being able to see beyond the moment

Uni-polar

A form of depression wherein one experiences periods of depression alternating with periods of wellness. A person with uni-polar mood disorder does not experience states of mania. (See the Introduction for more.)

Unwell

The term I use to describe myself when I am in a state of depression. I choose this word because it contains the positive word "well," and not the less positive word "ill."

Index of Pieces by Theme

Sometimes you may want to read an article or story on a particular topic or theme. Here is a list with twelve themes showing the articles and/or stories that are most pertinent to each.

Printed in the United States
2013